D0469233

O A R L

OXFORD AMERICAN RHEUMATOLOGY LIBRARY

Lupus

O A R L

OXFORD AMERICAN RHEUMATOLOGY LIBRARY

Lupus

The Essential Clinician's Guide

2nd Edition

Daniel J. Wallace, MD, FACP, FACR

Executive Series Editor,
Oxford American Rheumatology Library
Clinical Professor of Medicine
Division of Rheumatology
Cedars-Sinai Medical Center
David Geffen School of Medicine at UCLA
Los Angeles, California

OXFORD
UNIVERSITY PRESS

OXFORD
UNIVERSITY PRESS

Oxford University Press is a department of the University of Oxford.
It furthers the University's objective of excellence in research, scholarship,
and education by publishing worldwide.

Oxford   New York
Auckland   Cape Town   Dar es Salaam   Hong Kong   Karachi
Kuala Lumpur   Madrid   Melbourne   Mexico City   Nairobi
New Delhi   Shanghai   Taipei   Toronto

With offices in
Argentina   Austria   Brazil   Chile   Czech Republic   France   Greece
Guatemala   Hungary   Italy   Japan   Poland   Portugal   Singapore
South Korea   Switzerland   Thailand   Turkey   Ukraine   Vietnam

Oxford is a registered trademark of Oxford University Press
in the UK and certain other countries.

Published in the United States of America by
Oxford University Press
198 Madison Avenue, New York, NY 10016

© Oxford University Press 2014

Library of Congress Cataloging-in-Publication Data
Wallace, Daniel J. (Daniel Jeffrey), 1949– author.
Lupus : the essential clinician's guide/Daniel J. Wallace.—2nd edition.
    p. ; cm.—(Oxford American rheumatology library)
Includes bibliographical references and index.
ISBN 978–0–19–936196–0 (alk. paper)
I. Title.   II. Series: Oxford American rheumatology library.
[DNLM: 1. Lupus Erythematosus, Systemic. WD 380]
RC312.5.S5
616.7′72—dc23
2013031123

9 8 7 6 5 4 3 2 1
Printed in the United States of America
on acid-free paper

Contents

Chapter 1

The History of Lupus

Lupus (meaning "wolf" in Latin) was a Roman family name, and there was a St. Lupus who lived in central France in about A.D. 600.[1] How this name became connected with a disease is not known. Nevertheless, anecdotal case reports of what was probably the medical condition now called *lupus* appeared sporadically in writings from the tenth century on. Forms of cutaneous tuberculosis were also termed *lupus* in the early 1800s, and to this day, *lupus vulgaris* represents that condition. Several dermatological treatises in the 1830s and 1840s, particularly those by Pierre de Cazenave, provided illustrations and case presentations of what was certainly what is now known as lupus (Fig. 1.1).[2] Moritz Kaposi (for whom Kaposi's sarcoma is named) first used the description "discoid" to describe cutaneous lupus in the 1860s.

Credit for describing "disseminated," or systemic, lupus and connecting its rashes with organ involvement goes to Sir William Osler (1849–1919), who initially described our current concepts of the clinical aspects of the disease in three long articles published between 1872 and 1895.[3] Between 1900 and 1950, pathological descriptions of cardiac, pulmonary, and central nervous system involvement increased our general knowledge.

In 1941, Paul Klemperer coined the term "collagen vascular disorders" to apply to a group of what are now known to be autoimmune conditions. This led to initiatives to classify this family of disorders. The first criteria for systemic lupus erythematosus (SLE) were published in 1971, followed by revisions in 1981 and 1997, and a new classification in 2012. Other related variants of lupus, such as drug-induced lupus (1945), neonatal lupus (which is not actually lupus), overlap syndromes, mixed connective tissue disease, antiphospholipid syndrome (1983), and incomplete forms of lupus-like inflammation (undifferentiated connective tissue disease), followed. By the late 1970s, a nosological compilation of cutaneous manifestations of lupus was put together by James Gilliam.

Although a few cases of false-positive syphilis serologies were reported as early as 1909 in lupus patients, and hypergammaglobulinemia associated with lupus in 1943, the single major advance in identifying lupus by blood testing was published in 1949. Malcolm Hargraves, a hematologist at the Mayo Clinic, found "globular antibodies taking purple stain" in the marrow aspirate of a child with undiagnosed disease. The discovery of the "LE cell" greatly advanced the field, as it became possible for the first time for a blood test to be used to diagnose lupus, and biopsies were no longer mandatory. The LE cell turned out to be a DNA-histone nucleoprotein. Efforts to improve identification of protein markers in lupus resulted in antinuclear antibody and anti-DNA testing becoming available in the late 1950s. (Advances are summarized in Table 1.1.) Insights into

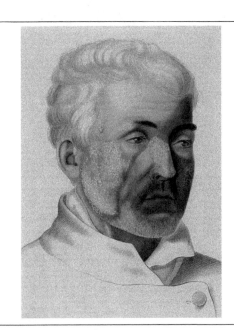

Figure 1.1 The first modern illustration of cutaneous lupus, labeled "lupus erythemateux" (1856). *Source:* Wallace DJ, Lyon I. Pierre Cazenave and the first detailed modern description of lupus erythemotosus. *Semin Arthritis Rheum.* 1999;28:305–313. Reprinted with permission, Elsevier, 1999.

Table 1.1 First descriptions of components of lupus

Description	Year	Author
Butterfly rash	1845	von Hebra
Arthralgia, adenopathy	1872	Kaposi
Nephritis, purpura	1895	Osler
Psychosis	1896	Bowen
Raynaud's phenomenon	1908	MacLeod
Biological false-positive syphilis serology	1909	Reinhart
Endocarditis	1923	Libman and Sacks
Hematoxylin bodies	1932	Gross
"Wire loop" glomeruli	1935	Baehr
Hyperglobulinemia	1943	Coburn and Moore
LE cell	1949	Hargraves
Lupus anticoagulant	1952	Conley and Hartman
Antinuclear antibody	1954	Miescher and Fauconnet
Anti-DNA	1957	Ceppillini and Robbins
Classification criteria	1971	Cohen and committee
Antiphospholipid syndrome	1983	Hughes, Harris, Asherson

the role of complement in inflammation and advances in immune techniques allowed anti-Sm, anti-RNP, anti-ENA, anti-Ro (SSA), and anti-La (SSB) to be identified and elucidated in the 1960s.

The first lupus clinic in the United States was started by Marian Ropes in Boston in 1922; her treatment armamentarium included aspirin and dermatologicals. The new availability of nitrogen mustard in 1947 and corticosteroids in 1948 revolutionized the treatment of SLE and raised the 50% five-year survival rate in 1948 to the current rate of 90% or better.

References

1. Benedek TG. Historical background of discoid and systemic lupus erythematosus. In: DJ Wallace and BH Hahn, eds. *Dubois' Lupus Erythematosus*. 7th ed. Philadelphia, PA: Lippincott Williams & Wilkins; 2007:2–15.

2. Hargraves MM. Production in vitro of the LE cell phenomenon: use of normal bone marrow elements and blood plasma from patients with acute disseminated lupus erythematosus. *Proc Staff Mayo Clin*. 1949;24:234–237.

3. Osler W. On the visceral complications of erythema exudativum multiforme. *Am J Med Sci*. 1895;110:629–646.

Chapter 2

Definitions and Classification

Systemic Lupus Erythematosus

Systemic lupus erythematosus (SLE) is a multisystem, pleomorphic disease in which inflammation, antibody production, and complement-fixing immune complex deposition result in tissue damage. Some regard it as a syndrome in that many patients have only a few aspects of the process (e.g., nephritis, thrombocytopenia) and are otherwise healthy and normal. In 1971, the American Rheumatism Association (forerunner of the American College of Rheumatology [ACR]) published preliminary criteria for the classification of SLE for clinical trials and population studies rather than for diagnostic purposes. Updated three times since, this definition has evolved as new insights and auto-antibodies have become known. Nevertheless, it appears that SLE is part of a spectrum of lupus-associated disorders. This section will attempt to categorize and define these subsets. The breakdown of different types of lupus is shown in Table 2.1.

The last revision of the ACR criteria (Table 2.2) defines SLE as being in-clusive of four cutaneous, four systemic, and three laboratory components. Four of the 11 are required for a diagnosis.[1] The 1997 criteria are over 90% sensitive and specific but have several inherent weaknesses: (1) many patients with biopsy-documented lupus nephritis do not meet the criteria; (2) the central nervous system definition has been made obsolete as advances in imaging, serological, and cerebrospinal fluid testing have become available; (3) issues of ANA-negative lupus are not adequately addressed; and (4) one can have cuta-neous lupus without systemic features and still fulfill the criteria. The Systemic Lupus International Collaborative Clinics (SLICC) proposed new criteria in 2012 to address these concerns. As sensitive and specific as the ACR criteria, for research studies and epidemiological surveys, either classification system can be used (Table 2.2b).

Cutaneous Lupus

Chronic cutaneous lupus erythematosus (CCLE; formerly known as *discoid lupus*) accounts for an overwhelming majority of cases of cutaneous lupus.[2] Although many CCLE patients have SLE, pure CCLE is defined by a biopsy demonstrating pathological changes consistent with the disorder in someone who does not fulfill the ACR criteria for SLE. Approximately half of all lupus is pure cutaneous; determining its true prevalence is difficult because many

Table 2.1 Types of lupus erythematosus

Cutaneous lupus, 40%

• Chronic cutaneous lupus erythematosus is 90% of this grouping

Systemic lupus erythematosus (SLE), 50%

• Organ-threatening disease, 25%

• Non-organ-threatening disease, 25%

Overlap syndrome/mixed connective tissue disease, 10% (involves fulfilling criteria for SLE and another rheumatic disease)

Drug-induced lupus erythematosus, <1%Neonatal Lupus,<1%

Table 2.2 The 1982/1997 American College of Rheumatology revised criteria for the classification of systemic lupus erythematosus

Cutaneous

1. Malar rash: fixed malar erythema, flat or raised

2. Discoid rash: erythematous-raised patches with keratic scaling and follicular plugging; atrophic scarring may occur

3. Photosensitivity: skin rash as an unusual reaction to sunlight; diagnosed by patient history or physician observation

4. Oral ulcers: oral or nasopharyngeal ulcers, usually painless; observed by physician

Systemic

1. Arthritis: non-erosive, involving two or more peripheral joints; characterized by tenderness, swelling, effusion

2. Serositis: pleuritis (convincing history of pleuritic pain or rub heard by physician, or evidence of pleural effusion) or pericarditis (documented by electrocardiogram, rub, or evidence of pericardial effusion)

3. Renal disorder: persistent proteinuria (>0.5 g/day or >3+) or cellular casts of any type

4. Neurological disorder: seizures or psychosis in the absence of other causes

Laboratory

1. Hematological disorder: hemolytic anemia or leukopenia (<4000 on two occasions), lymphopenia (<1500 on two occasions), or thrombocytopenia (<100,000 in the absence of offending drugs)

2. Immunological disorder: anti-ds DNA, or anti-Sm, or antiphospholipid antibodies (abnormal IgM or IgG anticardiolipin antibody, lupus anticoagulant, or false-positive syphilis serology)

3. Antinuclear antibody in the absence of drugs known to be associated with the "drug-induced lupus syndrome"

For identifying patients in clinical studies, a person shall be said to have SLE if any four or more of the 11 criteria are present either serially or simultaneously, during any interval of observation.

of these patients never see a rheumatologist and are managed by dermatologists; they are rarely hospitalized, as a person is not likely to die from a "rash." Gilliam's classification of lupus, put forth in the late 1970s, has been modified by some more recent advances, shown in Table 2.3.

Table 2.2b SLICC (Systemic Lupus Erythematosus International Collaborating Clinics) Classification For SLE

I. Biopsy documented nephritis excluding other causes, OR

II. One clinical and one immunological criterion from those listed below

  A. Clinical criteria in the absence of other causes:

     1. Acute cutaneous rash (malar, sun-sensitive, maculopapular, toxic epidermal necrolysis variant)

     2. Chronic cutaneous lupus (discoid, hypertrophic, profundus, tumidus, chilblains, mucosal, lichenoid)

     3. Oral ulcers (buccal, tongue, or nasal)

     4. Non-scarring alopecia

     5. Non-erosive inflammatory arthritis

     6. Serositis (pleural, pericardial)

     7. >0.5 G/day equivalent proteinuria or red blood cell urinary casts

     8. Neurological (seizures, psychosis, mononeuritis multiplex, myelitis, peripheral/cranial neuropathy, acute confusional state)

     9. Hemolytic anemia

    10. Leukopenia (<4K) or lymphopenia (<1K)

    11. Thrombocytopenia (<100 K)

  B. Immunological criteria:

     1. Antinuclear antibody present above reference range

     2. Anti double-stranded DNA >2 times reference range

     3. Antiphospholipid antibody (lupus anticoagulant, false-positive syphilis serology, anticardiolipin antibody >twice normal range, or anti beta-2 glycoprotein)

     4. Anti Sm

     5. Low C3, C4, or CH50 (total hemolytic complement)

     6. Positive direct Coombs without hemolytic anemia

Petri MA, Orbai AM, Alarcon GS, et al. Derivation and validation of the SLICC Classification Criteria for SLE. *Arthritis Rheum.* 2012;64:2677–2686.[6]

Table 2.3 Modified Gilliam classification for histologically specific lupus erythematosus–associated skin lesions

1. Acute cutaneous lupus: localized or generalized

2. Subacute cutaneous lupus: annular papulosquamous

3. Chronic cutaneous lupus: classical discoid lupus (localized or generalized), hypertrophic (verrucous), lupus profundus (panniculitis), mucosal lupus, lupus tumidus, toxic epidermal necrolysis, chilblains lupus (perniotic LE)

Neonatal Lupus

This rare condition occurs when a child of a mother who is anti-Ro (SSA) positive is born with a transient lupus rash that lasts several weeks before disappearing (the baby cannot make anti-Ro) or has congenital heart block. One anti-Ro-positive mother in 14 has a child with a rash; 2% of children born to these mothers have cardiac complications. It is not true lupus.

Drug-Induced Lupus Erythematosus

Approximately 15,000 cases of drug-induced lupus erythematosus (DILE) are reported annually in the United States. They do not generally fulfill the ACR criteria for SLE. Over 80 offending agents can induce DILE; 99% of cases disappear within three months of withdrawing the offending agent.

Mixed Connective Tissue Disease

One patient in 20 who fulfill criteria for SLE has Raynaud's phenomenon, an antibody to RNP (ribonucleoprotein), and also satisfies the ACR criteria for scleroderma, rheumatoid arthritis, or inflammatory myositis.[3] Once thought to have a benign condition, mixed connective tissue disease (MCTD) patients have a high prevalence of pulmonary hypertension and a poorer prognosis. A classification system is shown in Table 2.4.

Crossover and Overlap Syndromes

Individuals who do not have antibodies to anti-RNP but who have SLE and fulfill criteria for another rheumatic inflammatory disorder are thought to have a crossover or overlap syndrome. The prognosis is superior to that of MCTD.

Undifferentiated Connective Tissue Disease

For every patient with SLE, there are six or seven who display lupus-like symptoms without meeting SLE criteria. The presence of a positive antinuclear antibody or rheumatoid factor with certain inflammatory or vasculopathy features (e.g., Raynaud's phenomenon) is consistent with an undifferentiated connective tissue disease (UCTD).[4] One patient in three with a UCTD has spontaneous resolution of the process, one-third continue to have UCTD, and for one-third the disease will evolve into rheumatoid arthritis or SLE. Palindromic rheumatism also falls into this category. There is some evidence that hydroxychloroquine can prevent UCTD from progressing (Table 2.5).[5]

Table 2.4 Criteria for mixed connective tissue disease
Clinical criteria: Three of the following must be present: synovitis OR myositis (one must be present), hand edema, Raynaud's, acral sclerosis
AND
Serological criteria:
Positive anti-RNP into at least a moderate titer

Table 2.5 Criteria for undifferentiated connective tissue disease

1. Mandatory: inflammatory arthritis in >1 joint, OR Raynaud's, OR keratoconjunctivitis sicca
2. Mandatory: positive antinuclear antibody, rheumatoid factor, or anti-CCP
3. Need three of the following: myalgias, autoimmune rash, serositis, persistent fever without infection, adenopathy, elevated sedimentation rate or C-reactive protein, antiphospholipid antibody

Table 2.6 Criteria for the classification of the antiphospholipid syndrome

Clinical criteria:
- Vascular thrombosis: one or more episodes within 5 years
- Pregnancy morbidity: one or more unexplained deaths of a morphologically normal fetus after at least 10 weeks of gestation; OR before the 34th week of gestation due to preeclampsia, eclampsia, or placental insufficiency; OR 3 or more unexplained spontaneous abortions before the 10th week of gestation

Laboratory criteria:
- IgG or IgM isotype anticardiolipin antibodies on two occasions at least 3 months apart
- Lupus anticoagulant on two occasions at least 6 weeks apart
- Antibodies to β_2-glycoprotein (IgG or IgM isotypes) on two occasions 12 weeks apart

One clinical criterion plus one laboratory criterion must be present

Antiphospholipid Syndrome

One-third of persons with SLE have antiphospholipid antibodies; one-third of these (or about 11% of persons with SLE) sustain thromboembolic events or recurrent miscarriages as a consequence. The revised definition for antiphospholipid syndrome (APS) is presented in Table 2.6. One percent of persons with APS have recurrent thromboembolic episodes despite adequate therapy. This is referred to as catastrophic antiphospholipid syndrome (CAPS).

References

1. Hochberg MC. Updating the American College of Rheumatology revised criteria for the classification of systemic lupus erythematosus. *Arthritis Rheum.* 1997;40:1725.

2. Gilliam JN, Sontheimer RD. Skin manifestations of SLE. *Clin Rheum Dis.* 1982;8:207–218.

3. Alarcon-Segovia D, Cardiel MH. Comparison between 3 diagnostic criteria for mixed connective tissue disease. Study of 593 patients. *J Rheumatol.* 1989;16:328–334.

4. Alarcon GS, Williams GV, Singer JZ, et al. Early undifferentiated connective tissue disease. I. Early clinical manifestation in a large cohort of patients with undifferentiated connective tissue diseases compared with cohorts of well established connective tissue disease. *J Rheumatol.* 1991;18:1332–1339.

5. Miyakis S, Lockshin MD, Atsumi T, et al. International consensus on an update of the classification criteria for definite antiphospholipid syndrome (APS). *J Thromb Haemost.* 2006;4:295–306.

6. Petri MA, Orbai AM, Alarcon GS, et al. Derivation and validation of the SLICC Classification Criteria for SLE. *Arthritis Rheum.* 2012;64:2677–2686.

Chapter 3

Epidemiology of Systemic Lupus Erythematosus

Based on the definitions of lupus given in Chapter 2, 50% of all cases of lupus are systemic lupus erythematosus, evenly divided into organ-threatening (25%) and non–organ-threatening (25%) categories. The remainder of cases are cutaneous lupus (40%), mixed connective tissue disease and/or overlap syndromes (10%), and drug-induced lupus (<1%). There are seven undifferentiated connective tissue disease patients for every lupus patient. The true incidence and prevalence of systemic lupus in the United States are difficult to ascertain. Surveys have shown that only one in three patients told by a physician that he or she has SLE meets the American College of Rheumatology criteria.[1] Hospital discharge summaries may or may not list lupus as a comorbidity. Only 10,000 death certificates in the United States included lupus in a recent year, but these documents vary from state to state and are not configured to determine whether conditions such as lupus are present, concentrating instead upon the immediate cause of death. To avoid higher premiums, patients may not list lupus as a diagnosis on insurance forms, and many lupus patients do not have health insurance. There is wide variance relative to racial, ethnic, and geographic factors. Overall, the worldwide prevalence of lupus ranges from 14 to 172 cases per 100,000 people, and its annual incidence is 1.8 to 7.6 cases per 100,000.[2]

It has been estimated that as few as 300,000 and as many as 2 million individuals in the United States have SLE.[3] Lupus is the second or third most common rheumatic autoimmune disorder (Table 3.1).

Ethnicity

Approximately one white male in 10,000, one white female in 1,000, and one African American female in 250 in the United States have SLE.[4] People of color are diagnosed with lupus more frequently than are Caucasians, but this statistic can get complicated. For example, Filipinos and Chinese are diagnosed with lupus much more frequently than are Japanese or Malays. The highest rates of SLE have been reported among Afro-Caribbeans and Sioux Native Americans, but quality studies are lacking in the latter group. Lupus is relatively infrequent on the African continent.

Sex

Nearly 90% of persons with SLE are female, as opposed to 80% with chronic cutaneous lupus and 50% with drug-induced lupus. Most develop the disorder

Table 3.1 Principal epidemiological features of lupus erythematosus

1. Fifty percent of lupus is systemic lupus erythematosus (SLE), 40% is purely cutaneous lupus, 10% is crossover syndrome and/or mixed connective tissue disease, <1% is drug-induced lupus.

2. The prevalence of SLE averages 1 per 1000 adults, with subsets ranging from 1 per 250 African American women to 1 Caucasian male per 10,000 people.

3. Only 1 person in 3 in the United States told by their physician that they have lupus fulfills the American College of Rheumatology criteria for SLE. There are 7 cases of undifferentiated connective tissue disease for each true case of SLE.

during their reproductive years. The female-to-male ratio is 2:1 before puberty, as high as 8:1 during years of active menstruation, and 2.3:1 for patients over the age of 60 (Table 3.2).

Age

Children as young as several months old have been diagnosed with SLE, but fewer than 5% of lupus patients are prepubertal. Children tend to have more organ-threatening disease, but mortality rates are surprisingly low. Lupus developing in patients over the age of 50 tends to be less organ-threatening in nature and characterized by prominent musculoskeletal complaints, and it runs a blander course.

Trends

Recent surveys have suggested that the prevalence of SLE is modestly increasing. Whether or not this represents a true trend, or is simply the result of methods of ascertainment and availability of additional autoantibodies leading to the diagnosis of more difficult cases, has not been resolved.[5,6]

Table 3.2 Sex ratios at age of onset or at first diagnosis of systemic lupus erythematosus[7]

Age (y)	Female-to-male ratio
0–4	1.4:1
5–9	2.3:1
10–14	5.8:1
15–19	5.4:1
20–29	7.5:1
30–39	8.1:1
40–49	5.2:1
50–59	3.9:1
60–69	2.2:1

References

1. Hochberg MC, Perlmutter DL, Medsger TA, et al. Prevalence of self-reported, physician-diagnosed systemic lupus erythematosus in the USA. *Lupus*. 1995;4:454–456.

2. Rus V, Maury EE, Hochberg MC. The epidemiology of lupus. In: DJ Wallace and BH Hahn, eds. *Dubois' Lupus Erythematosus*. 7th ed. Philadelphia, PA: Lippincott Williams & Wilkins; 2007:34–44.

3. Lawrence RC, Helmick CG, Arnett FC, et al. Estimates of the prevalence of arthritis and selected musculoskeletal disorders in the United States. *Arthritis Rheum*. 1998;41:778–779.

4. Fessel WJ. Systemic lupus in the community. Incidence, prevalence, outcome and first symptoms; the high prevalence in black women. *Arch Intern Med*. 1974;134: 1027–1035.

5. Uramoto KM, Michet CJ Jr, Thumboo J, et al. Trends in the incidence and mortality of systemic lupus erythematosus, 1950–1992. *Arthritis Rheum*. 1999;42:46–50.

6. Lim SS, Drenkard C. The epidemiology of lupus. In: DJ Wallace and BH Hahn Eds. *Dubois' Lupus Erythematosus and Related Syndromes*. 8th ed. Philadelphia. Elsevier; 2013:8–24.

7. Masi AT, Kaslow RA. Sex effects in SLE: A clue to pathogenesis. *Arthritis Rheum*. 1978;21:480–484.

Chapter 4

Pathogenesis

Lupus is brought on when predisposing genetic factors activated by environmental factors, drugs, or infectious agents result in an abnormal immune response. This occurs when suppressor T cells fail to suppress, there are defects in cell signaling, there are defects in immune tolerance, apoptotic cells promote the creation of autoantibodies, and/or there is loss of regulatory cells that control autoreactivity. The latter results in the proliferation of B cells, leading to the formation of autoantibodies and immune complexes, which promote inflammation and tissue damage. Pathogenesis undergoes an often-gradual process consisting of several phases: predisposition, benign autoimmunity, prodrome, and clinical systemic lupus erythematosus. Only one person in 10 who possess lupus susceptibility genes ever develops full-blown lupus. Many individuals have "subclinical autoimmunity," or undifferentiated connective tissue disorders where the process is attenuated.

Phase 1: Predisposition

Genetic Predisposing Factors
Unlike with cystic fibrosis, for example, there is no single lupus gene. It is a polygenic disorder. At least 30 susceptibility genes for SLE have been identified, and their presence varies widely depending on race, ethnicity, and geography.[1] Genome scanning has shown that at least eight different chromosomal regions (especially on chromosome 1) contain susceptibility genes, especially in the presence of SSA or SSB. The risk for SLE is tenfold increased in monozygotic (identical) twins compared to dizygotic ones, and eight- to twentyfold in siblings of SLE patients compared to the healthy population. Most of the lupus-associated genes have odds ratios (relative risks) of less than 2.5 (1 would indicate no predisposition), and they are only of minimal clinical value. They predispose to autoimmunity because they determine which peptides can be presented to T-lymphocytes to activate help for autoantibody production and T-mediated immune responses. A handful of non-human leukocyte antigen (HLA) genes (e.g., C1q deficiency, DNAse, Trex1 mutations) have an odds ratio of 2.5 or greater, but are infrequently found. Other genes may be protective of lupus (e.g., a Toll-like receptor 5 [TLR5] polymorphism).

Epigenetics
Epigenetics refers to inherited or acquired modification of DNA without any changes in the DNA base sequence. These alterations occur via three mechanisms: DNA methylation, histone deacetylation, and microRNA. SLE is associated with hypomethylation, which leads to upregulated expression of surface molecules and T cell autoreactivity. Lupus-inducing drugs, ultraviolet light, and

microRNA can promote hypomethylation. Alterations in histones conformationally influence DNA transcription and repair. Deacetylation promotes autoimmunity and alters DNA signaling. Agents that interfere with this pathway are in clinical trials for a variety of autoimmune disorders. MicroRNA (miRNA) are non-coding small RNAs (19–25 nucleotides in length) "gene silencing" sequences that regulate gene expression at post-transcriptional levels. Over 1000 have been described in humans.

The Influence of Gender

Given that 90% of lupus patients are female, hormones certainly play a role. Estrogens are thought to be permissive for autoimmunity, and androgens protective (although males with lupus usually have more severe disease). Estradiol prolongs the life of autoreactive B and T-lymphocytes. After childbirth, women may be exposed to a graft-versus-host reaction from their fetuses (microchimerism), and their inactive X chromosome is enriched with hypomethylated genes (which can promote autoimmunity). A woman with lupus has a 2% risk of her son and a 10% risk of her daughter having lupus.

The Influence of the Environment

Ultraviolet light from the sun alters the structure of the dermis, which renders it more immunogenic, and kills skin cells, which induces apoptosis in keratinocytes (skin cells) and the formation of self antigen (Fig. 4.1). As only 28% of monozygotic twins both have SLE, environmental factors clearly play a role. Noninfectious agents associated with lupus include silica exposure; tobacco smoke; and possibly certain hair dyes, pesticides, allergens, foods, heavy metals, and solvents. Other than silica dust exposure (e.g., sandblasters, uranium mines) predisposing one to SLE, no other environmental agent, vocation, or other exposures have been proven to induce lupus.

Emotional stress clearly alters the immune system, and lupus has been infrequently temporally associated with routine vaccinations.

The Role of Infections

Lupus is often reported after a patient is subjected to an infectious process. Bacterial DNA serves as an adjuvant that can induce immune reactivity, and lupus patients have increased antibodies to retroviruses and viruses in the Epstein-Barr family. Molecular mimicry is thought to play a role in the process (e.g., a sequence of the Ro particle is similar to the Epstein-Barr nuclear antigen 1). There have been instances of lupus being "turned on" after a parvovirus B19 infection as well as other microbes. Infections can also cause a flare-up of preexisting lupus.

The Role of Drugs

Pharmaceuticals have multifaceted actions ranging from exacerbating or aggravating an immune process, to inducing lupus. For example, a drug can alter DNA or render it immunogenic and lead to the production of autoantibodies (e.g., procainamide). Other agents promote autoreactive T or B-lymphocytes (e.g., phenytoin). Hypomethylation of DNA results in altered DNA repair and autoantibody formation (e.g., fludarabine). Oxidized metabolites of certain agents in slow acetylators, for example, can induce an immune reaction (e.g.,

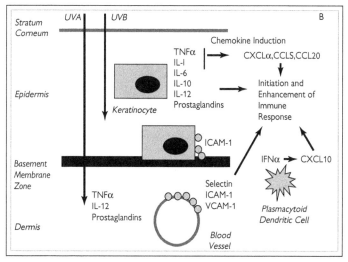

Figure 4.1 The role of ultraviolet light in lupus. *Key:* ICAM, intracellular adhesion molecule; IL, interleukin; TNF, tumor necrosis factor; UVA, ultraviolet A; UVB, ultraviolet B; VCAM, vascular cell adhesion molecule. *Source:* Wallace DJ, Hahn BH. *Dubois' Lupus Erythematosus,* 7th ed. Philadelphia, PA: Lippincott Williams & Wilkins; 2007. Reprinted with permission.

hydralazine, isonaizid). Certain drugs are sun-sensitizing (e.g., nonarylamine sulfa antibiotics, phenothiazines) and lead to a phototoxic inflammatory response. This sequence is summarized in Figure 4.2.

Phase 2: Benign Autoimmunity

A study of U.S. Army recruits showed that lupus autoantibodies are present for up to nine years in as many as 85% of patients before clinical lupus is evident.[2]

The development of autoantibodies precedes the first symptoms of SLE by two to nine years. Antinuclear antibodies first form, followed by anti DNA, antiphospholipid antibodies, and finally antibodies to Sm and RNP. These autoantibodies are self-perpetuating where amino acid sequences are T cell determinants and peptides activate helper T cells, and ultimately antibodies are formed. Antigen-antibody combinations (immune complexes) become bound by complement receptors and Fc Receptorscyto (FcR) receptors on immunoglobulins and become fixed in tissue where inflammation ensues.

Phase 3: Prodrome—the Innate Immune System and Loss of Tolerance in the Adaptive Immune System

At some point, the body's regulatory and tolerance systems are overwhelmed and patients begin to develop malaise and fatigue.[3] Two major immune networks contribute to the generation of autoreactive T cells and autoantibodies in

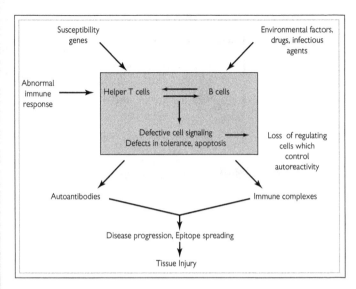

Figure 4.2 Factors promoting the development of systemic lupus erythematosus. *Source:* Wallace DJ. *The Lupus Book,* 5th ed. New York: Oxford University Press; 2012. Used with permission.

SLE: the innate immune system and the adaptive immune network.[4] Infections, self-antigens, and other danger signals activate the immune system via dendritic cells located in tissues that sample the environment (Fig. 4.3). Toll-like receptors (TLR) in dendritic cells recognize molecular patterns in bacteria and viruses. Cytosine phosphate Guianine (CpG) DNA sequences, which are common in bacterial DNA but uncommon in mammalian DNA, are bound by TLR7 and TLR9 in dendritic cells and B lymphocytes. Lupus dendritic cells may be activated, because many autoantigens have similar molecular patterns to microbial DNA. Binding of TLR7 and TLR9 in plasmacytic dendritic cells results in the release of α-interferon and other cytokines. It has been shown that lupus cells and tissue have increased expression of α-interferon (the "interferon signature").

Normal cells die via a mechanism known as *apoptosis.* Sometimes, debris from these dying cells becomes antigenic itself (e.g., nucleosomes, Ro in surface blebs, phosphatidyl serine in the outer cell membranes) which under the influence of oxidation, microorganisms, phosphorylation, and cleavage are processed by antigen-presenting cells. In the innate immune system, they are activated by DNA and RNA proteins complexed with TLR Toll via a process known as *NETosis* (neutrophil extracellular traps), which traps them and activates dendritic cells, cytokines, and interferon. The consequence of this is that effector T cells activate B cells (including plasmablasts) and form autoantibodies that deposit immunoglobulin and fix complement in tissues and promote inflammation. A similar pathway is initiated in adaptive immune responses.

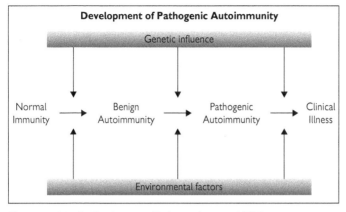

Figure 4.3 Arbuckle, Development of Pathogenic Immunity, *NEJM*[2]

The adaptive immune body's system of tolerance is lost via failed elimination of antigenic reactive lymphocytes in the spleen, lymph nodes, and bone marrow through inappropriate clonal deletion, receptor editing, or passive transfer. These mechanisms inhibit, delete, suppress, or ignore, which results in autoreactive cells that, when left untreated, can "break through." The persistence of debris from damaged cells (apoptosis) further leads to autoantibody formation. The deposition of immune complexes and failure to adequately clear them produces damage from the activation of complement and other mediators of inflammation (e.g., chemotaxis for lymphocytes and phagocytic cells, cytokines, chemokines, proteolytic enzymes; see Fig. 4.4).

Phase 4: Sustaining Clinical Lupus—the Adaptive Immune System and Loss of Immune Regulation

Immune complexes and apoptotic cells circulate in the bloodstream and need to be disposed of so they do not settle in tissues (which causes inflammation) or release chemicals (e.g., cytokines, chemokines) which also promote inflammation. In SLE, this clearance fails due to a variety of mechanisms: defective phagocytosis, altered transport by complement receptors, defective regulation of T helper cells by regulatory T cells, inadequate production or function of regulatory cells that kill or suppress autoreactive B cells, low production of interleukin 2 by T cells, and defects in apoptosis that permit the survival of effector T and autoreactive B cells (Fig. 4.5). When activated, T and B cells produce cytokines and autoantibodies. When underactivated, cells fail to undergo apoptosis, and B and T cells become autoreactive. Both phenomena occur in lupus. Defects in immune tolerance permit prolonged survival of B and T cells, which leads to activated B cells, memory B cells, and plasma cell formation, and ultimately autoreactive B cells. These are further influenced by B cell surface antigen receptors, soluble BlyS (B lymphocyte

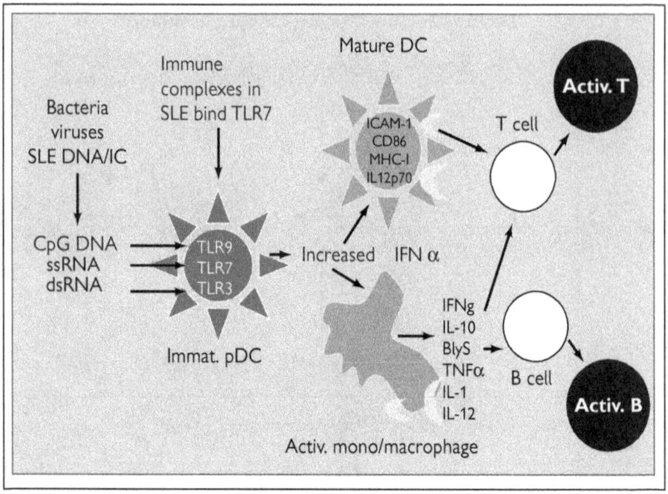

Figure 4.4 Innate immune response in systemic lupus erythematosus (SLE). *Key:* DC, dendritic cells; IFNα, interferon alpha; IL, interleukin; ICAM, intracellular adhesion molecule; MHC, major histocompatibility complex; TLR, Toll-like receptor. Reprinted with permission.

stimulation—which is what is blocked by the drug belimumab), genetic polymorphisms (variations) affecting B cell receptor signaling, and the intracellular mobilization of calcium. Regulatory T cells (T reg) suppress inflammation, and their function is diminished in lupus. T cell receptor activation is altered, and T reg mechanisms fail, which allow the activation of the pro-inflammatory cytokine interleukin-17. When there is a defect in T suppressor apoptosis, autoreactive B cells form.

Phase 5: Tissue Damage

Tissue damage is produced by the deposition of circulating immune complexes into tissue, which in turn activates endothelial cells, cytokines, and chemokines. In the kidneys, this produces inflammation, followed by proliferation and ultimately fibrosis (scarring). Complement activation, overloading of the Complement Receptor 1 (CR1) transport system, antibodies to complement components (anti Complement 1 qC1q), and congenital or acquired deficiency in complement components also lead to tissue inflammation and damage. Lupus is also characterized by accelerated atherosclerosis. This results from circulating immune complexes and complement split products activating endothelial cells in coronary arteries, which leads to the release of chemokines, cytokines, and activated monocytes. A nidus of plaque forms, which, in combination with oxidized LDL (bad cholesterol), forms "foam" cells that produce damage to coronary arteries. Chronicity of this process results in tissue and organ damage (see Fig. 4.6).

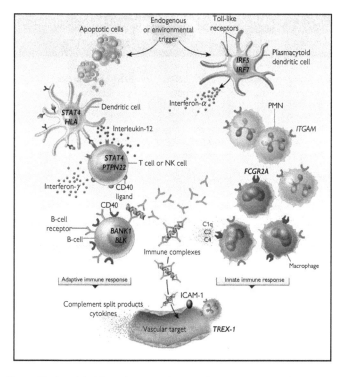

Figure 4.5 A model of the pathogenesis of systemic lupus erythematosus that implicates the products of disease-associated polymorphic genes. Crow, A Model of the Pathogenesis of SLE, *NEJM*[5]

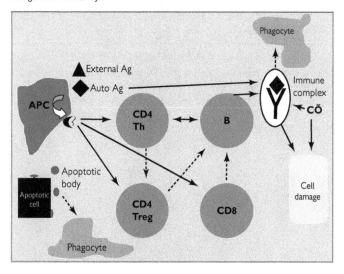

Figure 4.6 Adaptive immunity in systemic lupus erythematosus (SLE). *Key:* APC, anaphase-promoting complex; Ag, antigen. Reprinted with permission.

Table 4.1 Explanations for the development of systemic lupus erythematosus in genetically predisposed individuals with autoantibodies

1. Critical "dose" of susceptibility genes
2. Environment: infection, ultraviolet light, drugs, chemicals, hormones, stress
3. Antigens: alteration to more immunogenic forms, sustained exposure to high quantities of apoptotic cells, molecular mimicry, autoantigen-induced epitope spreading
4. Band T-cell abnormalities: activation with less antigen, more reactivity, abnormal receptor engagement, resistance to apoptosis, cytokine interactions
5. Pathogenic autoantibody subsets: based on charge, avidity, idiotypes, persistence of immune complexes
6. Targeted tissues more permissive to antibodies

Summary

When individuals with susceptibility genes are exposed to environmental factors, chemicals, certain microbes, or drugs, a milieu is created wherein the regulatory and suppressor T cells are overwhelmed and malfunction. Defects in tolerance, cell signaling, and apoptosis result in an increase in B cells and, ultimately, autoantibody formation. The inability of the reticuloendothelial system to adequately clear circulating immune complexes leads to further inflammation and the deposition of these complexes into tissue[5,6] (Table 4.1).

References

1. Croker JA, Kimberly RA. Genetics of susceptibility and severity in systemic lupus erythematosus. *Curr Opin Rheumatol.* 2005;17:529–537.

2. Arbuckle MR, McClain MT, Rubertone MB. Development of autoantibodies before the clinical onset of systemic lupus erythematosus. *N Engl J Med.* 2003;349:1526–1533.

3. Hahn BB, Ebling F, Singh RR, et al. Cellular and molecular mechanisms of autoantibody production in lupus. *Ann N Y Acad Sci.* 2005;115:40–417.

4. Christensen SR, Shlomchik MJ. Regulation of lupus-related autoantibody production and clinical disease by Toll-like receptors. *Semin Immunol.* 2007;19:11–23.

5. Crow MK. Collaboration, genetic associations and lupus erythematosus. *N Engl J Med.* 2008;358:956–961.

6. Tsokos GC. Systemic lupus erythematosus. *N Engl J Med.* 365;2110–2011.

Chapter 5

Clinical Symptoms and Signs

Lupus is known for its protean manifestations, which affect every organ system. These are identified via symptoms, signs, and laboratory or imaging abnormalities. This section reviews the principal complaints and physical findings associated with the disease (Table 5.1).[1]

Chief Complaint

Half of persons with systemic lupus erythematosus present with organ-threatening disease. The remaining individuals do not present with cardiopulmonary, hepatic, or renal symptoms; central nervous system (CNS) vasculitis; hemolytic anemia; or thrombocytopenia on initial evaluation. Organ involvement is relatively easy to diagnose—a chest radiograph, electrocardiogram, blood chemistry panel, complete blood count, and urinalysis usually point the physician in the correct direction. It takes a mean of three months from the onset of symptoms to diagnose these individuals. On the other hand, it can often take one to two years and several physician consultations before the presence of organ-sparing lupus is ascertained. Rashes can shorten the length to time of diagnosis, but young, healthy-appearing women with non-specific symptoms of fatigue and aching are often thought to have other processes or are given psychosocial explanations. A review of the chief complaint of new lupus patients revealed that the principal manifestations were arthralgia (62%) and cutaneous symptoms (especially newly discovered photosensitivity) (20%), followed by fever and malaise.

Constitutional Findings: Fever, Malaise, Fatigue, Anorexia, and Weight Loss

Constitutional complaints are generalized manifestations of the disease that do not fall into any organ-system category. They include fever, malaise, fatigue, anorexia, and weight loss.

The definition of *fever* is a temperature greater than 99.6°F. Low-grade fevers are often a presenting feature of SLE, and patients may not be aware of their elevated temperature. The usual source of nonfocal fever is untreated or undertreated inflammation. Often associated with tachycardia and relative hypotension, infection needs to be ruled out. Other causes of elevated temperature include medication reactions. Fevers need to be viewed seriously, especially if the patient is taking salicylates, nonsteroidal drugs, or corticosteroids that reduce body temperature.

Table 5.1 Approximate prevalence of selected symptoms, signs, and laboratory abnormalities of systemic lupus erythematosus during the course of the disease in the United States, based on a summation of findings in diverse cohorts	
Positive antinuclear antibody	97%
Malaise and fatigue	90%
Arthralgia, myalgia	90%
Sun sensitivity, skin changes	70%
Cognitive dysfunction	70%
Low C3 or C4 complement	61%
Fever due to lupus	57%
Antibodies to dsDNA	50%
Arthritis	50%
Leukopenia	46%
Pleuritis	44%
Anemia	42%
Alopecia	40%
Nephritis, proteinuria	40%
Anticardiolipin antibody	35%
Malar rash	35%
Central nervous system	32%
Increased gamma globulin	32%
Weight loss due to lupus	27%
Raynaud's	25%
Hypertension	25%
Sjögren's	25%
Oral ulcerations (mouth, nose)	20%
Discoid lesions	20%
Central nervous system vasculitis	15%
Adenopathy	15%
Pleural effusion	12%
Subacute cutaneous lupus	10%
Myositis	10%
Avascular necrosis	10%

Lupus patients complain of a sense of malaise and fatigue. Over 90% with the disease report this to their physician, and its lack of specificity can be problematic. Loss of stamina and endurance, aching or flu-like symptoms, and a sense of "not feeling right" or "having the blahs" are examples of descriptions that might be given to an examining physician. Infection, depression, anemia, hormonal imbalance, medication reactions, and stress need to be considered in the differential diagnosis.

Half of all lupus patients report a loss of appetite with resulting weight loss upon initial presentation. Ten percent note a 10% loss of body weight over a three-month period. This nonspecific finding usually does not occur later in the disease course, especially if the patient is taking corticosteroids. Lupus with nephrosis is also associated with labile weight alterations.

Cutaneous Manifestations

Photosensitivity

Two-thirds of lupus patients self-report sensitivity to sunlight.[2] Half of these (one-third of those with SLE) have reproducible rashes or a wheal-and-flare response when exposed to ultraviolet (UV) light in a controlled setting. Reactions range from a mild rash to fevers, malaise, adenopathy, arthritis, and severe rashes. Some patients have no problem going out in the sun; for others, it is dose- and time-related. UV exposure can be present on cloudy days and is greater at higher altitudes and midday. It is believed that UVA2 (320 to 340 nm) and UVB (340 to 400 nm) light are harmful in SLE; the UVA1 (290 to 320 nm) spectrum may actually have anti-inflammatory properties.

Malar (Butterfly) Rash

Present in a little more than one-third of lupus patients, the butterfly rash is one of the disease's most recognizable features. The malar eminence is so angled as to receive more UV exposure. The rash is often worse on the left side, as exposure can be greater from reflected light when driving a vehicle in sunny weather. It needs to be differentiated from rosacea (which spares the nasolabial folds but can coexist with lupus rashes) and polymorphous light eruption in fair-skinned individuals, among other lesions.

Mucocutaneous Lesions

Oral ulcers are present in 20% of patients with SLE and need to be distinguished from herpetic lesions (Fig. 5.1). Mostly located on the buccal mucosa and hard palate, and less frequently on the soft palate or tongue, the lesions often have a sharply marginated, irregularly scalloped white border and may be painless. Empiric treatment, herpes serologies, or, if necessary, a biopsy can help consolidate the diagnosis. Other inflammatory diseases, such as Behçet's, Crohn's, Wegener's, and reactive arthritis, are associated with oral ulcerations.

Alopecia (Hair Loss)

Hair thinning or loss is a common manifestation of SLE (Fig. 5.2). It can be due to inflammation; cutaneous, scarring scalp lesions; or medications such as immune-suppressive drugs or corticosteroids (which produce thinning in the male pattern of baldness). Lupus patients tend to have fine, downy, dry hair with increased fragility and may report clumps being shed after showering.

Changes in Pigmentation

Increased or decreased pigmentation is present in 10% of patients. Post-inflammatory changes and antimalarial therapies are responsible for most of this. A few patients have coexisting vitiligo. Corticosteroids may produce bruises, or ecchymoses.

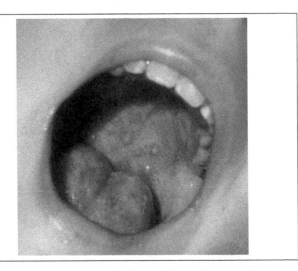

Figure 5.1 Oral ulcerations in patient with systemic lupus erythematosus. ©1972–2004 American College of Rheumatology Clinical Slide Collection. Used with permission.

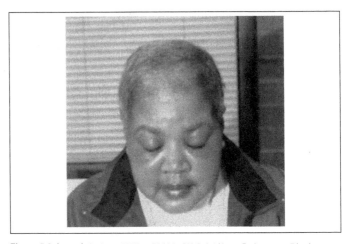

Figure 5.2 Lupus hair. *Source:* Wallace DJ, Hahn BH. *Dubois' Lupus Erythematosus,* 7th ed. Philadelphia, PA: Lippincott Williams & Wilkins; 2007. Reprinted with permission.

Hives and Urticaria

Seen in 10% of SLE patients, this pruritic reaction is known as "lupus urticaria." It may be found more frequently in atopic patients. Topical or systemic steroids, antihistamines, and H_2 blockers are useful; refractory cases are often responsive to a three-month course of cyclosporine.

Facial Telangiectasia

This is not a true form of lupus but is commonly seen among lupus patients who apply topical, fluorinated corticosteroids to the face, especially the cheeks, on a chronic basis. Cutaneous atrophy, cigarette-paper-thin skin, and dermal atrophy ensue, creating the appearance of small, capillary-like telangiectasias. Facial lupus rashes can be managed with the application of nonfluorinated hydrocortisone or immunophillin-binding agents (e.g., topical tacrolimus). Potent topical corticosteroids should never be used for longer than two weeks at a time.

Cutaneous Subsets Associated with Lupus Erythematosus

Acute Cutaneous Lupus

This can be a localized or generalized process that is almost always part of systemic lupus activity. Although it can be an isolated phenomenon after sun exposure, most patients have multisystem involvement and require more than topical therapy.

Subacute Cutaneous Lupus

Seen in 10% of patients with any form of lupus, this dermal reaction presents as a papulosquamous or annular lesion that is non-scarring (Fig. 5.3). Associated with anti-Ro (SSA), these lesions are more resistant to anti-malarial therapies and may respond to the addition of retinoid regimens and corticosteroids. Over 20 pharmaceutical agents can induce subacute cutaneous lupus (SCLE), particularly hydrochlorothiazide, angiotensin- converting enzyme inhibitors, calcium channel blockers, and terbinafine.

Chronic Cutaneous (Discoid) Lupus Erythematosus

This subset represents 10% of the lupus spectrum and is also observed in 20% of persons with SLE (Figs. 5.4 and 5.5). Usually appearing as a thick, plaque-like, adherent lesion in sun-exposed areas, chronic cutaneous (discoid) lupus erythematosus (CCLE) is histologically characterized by hyperkeratosis, follicular plugging, dermal atrophy, vacuolation, pigment changes, induration, and scarring. Basement membranes are thickened, and a lichenoid infiltrate and periappendageal inflammation are usually present. The transition rate of CCLE to SLE, if it is not present initially, is 15% over five years. Antimalarial therapies and topical regimens are usually quite effective. CCLE that appears only above the neck rarely disseminates.

Other Cutaneous Variants of Lupus

Lupus profundus is a rare form of cutaneous lupus (seen in 1 in every 200 patients), with lumpy lesions reflecting inflammatory lesions of the lower dermis and subcutaneous tissue. Exaggerated hyperkeratosis is termed *hypertrophic discoid lupus erythematosus.*

The presence of excessive dermal mucin in cutaneous lupus is known as *lupus erythematosus tumidus.* Reddish-purple patches with plaques on the fingers, toes, and face precipitated by cold, damp climates is called *lupus pernio,* or *chilblains. Bullous lupus* is a blistering variant of lupus with pemphigoid features. It is usually responsive to dapsone. *Calcinosis* is noted in a small number of patients, many of whom also have a scleroderma overlap (Table 5.2).

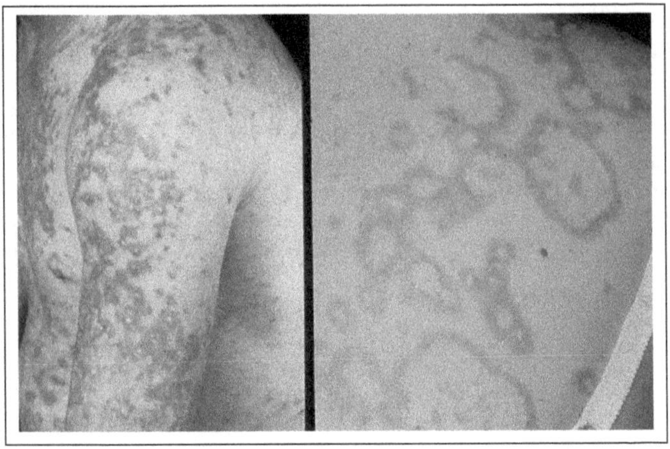

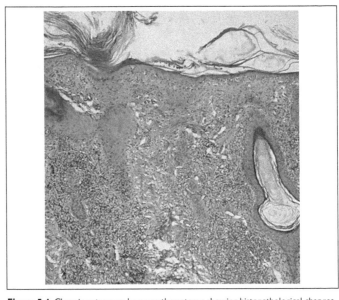

Figure 5.3 Subacute cutaneous lupus erythematosus. ©1972–2004 American College of Rheumatology Clinical Slide Collection. Used with permission.

Figure 5.4 Chronic cutaneous lupus erythematosus showing histopathological changes on skin biopsy and discoid lesions in a malar distribution. ©1972–2004 American College of Rheumatology Clinical Slide Collection. Used with permission.

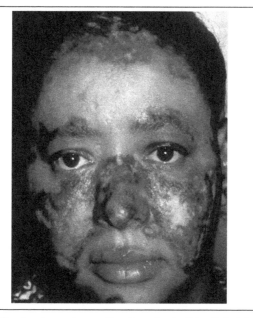

Figure 5.5 Chronic cutaneous lupus erythematosus showing histopathological changes on skin biopsy and discoid lesions in a malar distribution. ©1972–2004 American College of Rheumatology Clinical Slide Collection. Used with permission.

Cutaneovascular Manifestations

Cutaneous Vasculitis

Vasculitis in lupus is manifested by intimal proliferation, medial necrosis, and adventitial fibrosis. SLE usually affects the small and medium-sized arterioles, but leukocytoclastic vasculitis, hypersensistivity vasculitis, and cutaneous small-vessel vasculitis are present in the skin as well. The latter affects postcapillary venules and can present as palpable petechial areas on dependent areas. Cutaneous necrosis, ulceration, and gangrene occur infrequently (Fig. 5.6). Corticosteroids, colchicines, and dapsone may be useful in the treatment of cutaneous vasculitis. *Cryoglobulinemic vasculitis* has been reported in one lupus patient per 1,000. *Purpura* that is palpable may be associated with cutaneous vasculitis and should be differentiated from corticosteroid-induced ecchymosis.

Raynaud's Phenomenon

Raynaud's phenomenon in SLE represents a combination of intimal hyperplasia of the digital arterioles and autonomic-mediated vasomotor instability (Fig. 5.7). The latter promotes exaggerated vasodilatation with exposure to warmth and vasoconstriction with cold. This produces color changes in the digits, ranging from red to white to blue. Seen in 25% of persons with lupus, Raynaud's

Table 5.2 Cutaneous manifestations of lupus erythematosus
TYPES OF CUTANEOUS LUPUS
Acute cutaneous lupus erythematosus
Subacute cutaneous lupus erythematosus
Chronic (discoid) cutaneous lupus erythematosus
Lupus profundus
Hypertrophic lupus
Lupus tumidus
Lupus pernio (chilblains)
Bullous lupus
MANIFESTATIONS OF CUTANEOUS LUPUS
Sun sensitivity
Oral, nasal, or genital ulcerations
Butterfly rash
Hair loss or thinning
Changes in pigmentation
Hives or welts
Telangiectasias
Calcinosis
CUTANEO-VASCULAR MANIFESTIONS OF LUPUS
Cutaneous vasculitis
Cryoglobulinemic vasculitis
Raynaud's
Livedo reticularis
Erythromelalgia
Ulceration/gangrene
Purpura

phenomenon is often independent of disease activity, and more serious forms are associated with focal or periungual fingertip ulcerations, fingertip tuft atrophy, and gangrene. Overlap syndromes with scleroderma features and mixed connective tissue disease are found with more serious cases of Raynaud's phenomenon.

Other Cutaneovascular Manifestations

Livedeo reticularis is commonly observed in SLE and is statistically associated with the presence of antiphospholipid syndrome (termed *Sneddon's syndrome*). It represents a dysautonomia and appears as a net-like, blanchable red-purple ring in a lacelike, checkerboard pattern (Fig. 5.8). Livedo reticularis does not require treatment unless it is associated with a livedoid vasculitis, where the skin breaks down. *Erythromelalgia* is a burning pain of the hands and feet accompanied by macular edema and warmth. *Palmar erythema* is usually benign and is a reflection of autonomic instability. *Periungual telangiectasias* and *atrophie blanche* are seen in a small number of patients.

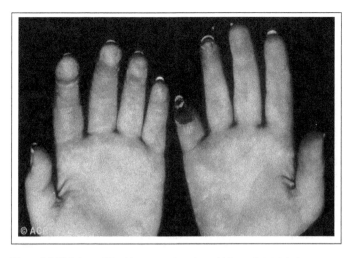

Figure 5.6 Digital vasculitis with gangrene in patient with lupus. ©1972–2004 American College of Rheumatology Clinical Slide Collection. Used with permission.

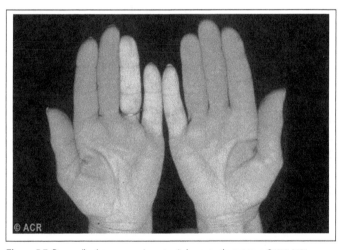

Figure 5.7 Raynaud's phenomenon in systemic lupus erythematosus. ©1972–2004 American College of Rheumatology Clinical Slide Collection. Used with permission.

Musculoskeletal Manifestations

Arthralgias and Arthritis

Arthralgias are present in at least 80% of SLE patients, whereas observable inflammatory arthritis involving two or more joints is found in 50% at some point in the course of the disease. Magnetic resonance imaging suggests a bland,

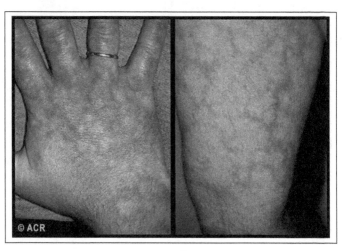

Figure 5.8 Livedo reticularis. ©1972–2004 American College of Rheumatology Clinical Slide Collection. Used with permission.

rheumatoid-like synovitis. Although 30% with SLE have a positive rheumatoid factor, only 10% with lupus have a rheumatoid-like arthritis. Fewer than 5% have radiographic erosions. Patients who have both rheumatoid arthritis and SLE are said to have "rhupus." Stiffness and aching are common; they are usually associated with a morning "gel" and joint pain and are bilateral and symmetrical in distribution, especially affecting the small joints of the hands and feet. Aspirated lupus synovial fluid has a white count of 2,000 to 15,000/mm³, consistent with a low-grade inflammatory process. Concurrent osteoarthritis is common in patients over the age of 40; 25% with SLE also meet the American College of Rheumatology (ACR) criteria for fibromyalgia. Deformity is common, but grip strength and function may be impaired. Synovitis also involves the tendons and bursae; rheumatoid nodules occur in less than 5% and are usually small and pea-sized. Lupus patients often demonstrate a Jaccoud's deformity, wherein the ulnar deviation at the metacarpal phalangeal joints is subluxable in that they can be manually straightened.[6]

Myalgias and Myositis

Myalgias are noted by 70% of lupus patients, but frank myositis raising muscle enzymes is observed in 5% to 10% during the disease process. Creatine phosphokinase levels rarely rise above 500 IU unless an overlap syndrome is present. Electromyograms confirm suspicions of a myopathic process. A several-weeks' course of medium-dose prednisone (20 to 40 mg/day) is usually salutary for muscle inflammation associated with lupus. The differential diagnosis mandates ruling out drug-induced myalgias/myositis (as with statin therapy), hypothyroidism, fibromyalgia, or viral infections (such as influenza or hepatitis). Long-term corticosteroid therapy induces type IIa fiber atrophy, which is difficult to reverse. Tapering of corticosteroid therapy can also induce a "steroid withdrawal" myalgia, which is usually managed with agents such as clonazepam or interventions to ensure optimal sleep architecture.

Osteopenia and Osteoporosis

Inflammation from active lupus and anti-inflammatory regimens such as corticosteroids and methotrexate are both associated with bone demineralization. The ACR recommends that any patient taking 5 mg of prednisone or more (or the equivalent) daily for longer than one month be receiving a bisphosphonate. It is prudent to measure bone densitometry every one to two years in high-risk individuals (e.g., Caucasians, smokers, those with thin body habitus or strong family history for osteoporosis). The use of calcium, vitamin D, hormonal interventions, calcitonin, bisphosphonates, or, if necessary, parathyroid hormone (parathormone) should be decided on a case-by-case basis.

Avascular Necrosis (Osteonecrosis)

One of the most feared complications of chronic corticosteroid therapy is avascular necrosis. Fatty clots produced by corticosteroids clog up the bone's blood supply and deprive it of oxygen. Infarcted bone is most commonly noted in the hip, but any joint can be involved. In 10% of cases, avascular necrosis is found in lupus patients who are not taking corticosteroids. Magnetic resonance imaging is the gold standard for identifying the process (Fig. 5.9). Early avascular necrosis of the hip can be treated with vascular grafting or core decompression, but most patients ultimately require joint replacement along with analgesic therapies.

Pulmonary Involvement

Pleurisy

Patients with lupus may complain of pain on taking a deep breath, shortness of breath, windedness, wheezing, or chest pains. The most common problem relates to pleurisy. At autopsy, most lupus patients show evidence of pleural scarring or prior inflammation. Manifested by pain or a catching sensation on taking a deep breath, pleural symptoms are present in 60% of lupus patients, and frank effusions noted in 25%, during a lifetime. Serosal surfaces frequently become inflamed in the condition; associated pericardial and peritoneal involvement is not uncommon. It is important to note that pleurisy is not considered organ-threatening; the parenchyma is not involved. Pleuritic discomfort can also be caused by an infection or environmental exposures. Chest radiographs are normal in most patients; pleural scarring is evident in some. In the absence of pleural fluid, pleuritis is managed with nonsteroidal drugs, antimalarials, and, if necessary, a short course of corticosteroids. Some patients with concurrent fibromyalgia have pleuritic-like complaints. Acute-phase reactants (e.g., sedimentation rate, C-reactive protein) can guide the practitioner as to how active the process is. Computed tomography scanning and ultrasonography may be necessary. If present, pleural fluid obtained at thoracentesis can be an exudate (suggestive of active inflammatory disease, malignancy, or infection) or a transudate (usually seen with concurrent nephrosis or pericarditis;[8] see Table 5.3).

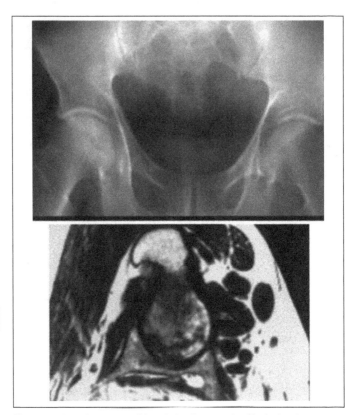

Figure 5.9 Avascular necrosis of the right hip shown on plain film (*top*) and T1-weighted magnetic resonance imaging (*bottom*). From Wallace DJ, Hahn BH. *Dubois' Lupus Erythematosus*, 7th ed. Philadelphia, PA: Lippincott Williams & Wilkins; 2007. Reprinted with permission.

Acute Lupus Pneumonitis

Seen in 1% to 9% of persons with SLE, patients with acute lupus pneumonitis (ALP) present acutely with shortness of breath and fever. Often treated telephonically as a pulmonary infection with antibiotics, the process progresses rapidly if high doses of corticosteroids are not prescribed. ALP manifests as an interstitial infiltrate containing neutrophils and immune complexes. Patients should promptly undergo bronchoscopy or a bronchoalveolar lavage. Cultures are negative. ALP has an 80% mortality rate if not diagnosed within two weeks of onset; recovery is usually rapid with appropriate treatment.

Interstitial Lung Disease

Unlike ALP, interstitial lung disease (ILD) is a chronic process, and many years often elapse without the patient's making any complaint. Most symptomatic patients describe being mildly short of breath or easily winded on exertion. Strongly associated with Sjögren's syndrome, mixed connective tissue disease,

Table 5.3 Pleural fluid in systemic lupus erythematosus
Transudate of exudates
Color: yellow to amber
Protein: >3g if exudate and pH >7.35
WBC: 3000 to 5000 cells/mL, monocyte and lymphocyte predominance
Glucose: near serum levels
ANA > serum titer, C3 and C4 decreased Sediment: LE cells on Wright stain

and overlap syndromes, ILD causes a lymphocytic infiltrate. Infection and lymphoproliferative processes need to be ruled out. Pulmonary-function testing demonstrates restrictive findings, and respirations can be rapid and shallow. The gold standard of diagnosis is a high-resolution computed tomography scan. A ground-glass appearance tends to suggest reversibility, while honeycombing goes against it. If the process is not scarred down, anti-inflammatory regimens are indicated. Respiratory failure is extremely uncommon.

Pulmonary Embolus

Almost all lupus patients who sustain a pulmonary embolus have antiphospholipid antibodies. Seen in 5% to 10% of lupus patients in their lifetime, pulmonary emboli present acutely with shortness of breath, chest pains, tachycardia, and low-grade fever. Thrombophlebitis may be evident. Oxygen saturations are decreased, and elevated D-dimer levels along with mismatching on a ventilation/perfusion lung scan usually confirm the diagnosis. Pulmonary emboli are managed with the same regimen of anticoagulation as is used in any non-lupus patient with this condition: heparin followed by warfarin. If antiphospholipid antibodies are present, lifelong warfarin may be advised, as the recurrence rate for thromboembolic disease is high.

Pulmonary Hemorrhage

Less than 1% of lupus patients experience bleeding into their air sacs, but this represents up to 10% of all lupus deaths. Usually of acute onset, patients appear ill and complain of hemoptysis along with evidence for multisystem activity. Suggested by alveolar infiltrates on chest radiography and confirmed at bronchoscopy by inflammation without infection and staining for immune complexes, pulmonary hemorrhage is managed with combination anti-inflammatory regimens (Fig. 5.10).

Pulmonary Hypertension

Most lupus patients who develop clinically significant elevations in pulmonary pressures have antiphospholipid syndrome (with recurrent pulmonary emboli), mixed connective tissue disease (anti-RNP positive), or a scleroderma overlap. The pathological stimulus is thought to be related to endothelial cell dysfunction with abnormal vascular responses. Complaints of breathlessness are common; chest radiographs may be normal. Pulmonary pressures are estimated with a 2-D Doppler echocardiogram and precisely quantitated at right-heart catheterization. Readings above 50 mm Hg are usually managed more aggressively, with approaches that will be reviewed in Chapter 11. The heretofore dismal prognosis for pulmonary hypertension is slowly improving, and heart/lung transplantation has led to some cures.

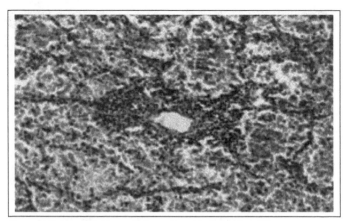

Figure 5.10 Hemosiderin granules in a patient with alveolar hemorrhage.

Shrinking Lung Syndrome

Elevated hemidiaphragms seen on chest radiographs are usually due to chronic pleural scarring and can result in shortness of breath. The condition is termed "shrinking lung syndrome." This rare manifestation may respond to corticosteroids and occasionally but infrequently necessitates pleural decortication.

Reversible Hypoxemia

Active disease is rarely associated with hypoxemia and hypocapnea with a wide alveolar-arterial gradient. Chest radiographs are normal. Inflammation or complement split products may play a role, and the process is responsive to corticosteroids.

The cardiopulmonary manifestations of SLE are summarized in Table 5.4.

Table 5.4 Prevalence of principal cardiopulmonary manifestations of systemic lupus erythematosus	
Pleuritic discomfort	60%
Myocardial dysfunction	40%
Hypertension	25%
Pleural effusion	25%
Pericardial effusion	25%
Interstitial lung disease	10%
Pulmonary embolus	7%
Acute lupus pneumonitis	5%
Pulmonary hypertension	5%
Libman-Sacks endocarditis	3%
Shrinking lung syndrome	1%
Pulmonary hemorrhage	1%

Cardiovascular Manifestations

A cardiac history may reveal chest pains, pressure, palpitations, or shortness of breath. The cardiac examination should include measuring pulse and blood pressure, pressing the chest wall for tenderness, and auscultation. Tachycardia can be a sign of inflammation or fever; it may be associated with relative hypotension. Dysautonomic responses (e.g., tilt-table testing) are not uncommon. The most common chest complaint in a lupus patient is chest pain. Costochondritis and gastroesophageal reflux disease (GERD) are typically the sources of this, with pericardial irritation frequently noted. Other causes include myocarditis or angina.[7]

The Pericardium

Pericardial involvement is found in 60% of lupus patients at autopsy and incidentally, and asymptomatically in 25% on 2-D echocardiogram. Frank effusions are seen in 25% during the course of disease but in fewer than 5% of patients at any given point in time. The effusions can be exudates (active inflammation) or transudates (as with concurrent nephrosis or ascites). Patients note a pressure-like discomfort relieved by leaning forward. Chronic inflammation leads to pericardial scarring, and individuals note ongoing pressure sensations.

The Myocardium: Myocarditis and Myocardial Dysfunction

Myocardial dysfunction (often from subclinical inflammation) is found on stress echocardiography in 40% with SLE, but only 5% to 10% ever experience frank myocarditis. Lupus myocarditis presents similarly to, and is often confused with, viral myocarditis. Patients complain of chest discomfort, cough, and dyspnea along with constitutional symptoms of extracardiac systemic inflammation. Concurrent features may include angina pectoris (classical), microvascular angina (small vessel disease, or "Raynaud's of the heart") and elevated muscle enzymes. The diagnosis is solidified by traditional angiography, a 64-slice computed tomography "virtual angiogram," or myocardial biopsy. Although congestive heart failure (CHF) was common 40 to 50 years ago, only a small percentage of lupus patients with significant myocardial dysfunction ever evolve to this point now. Brought on or aggravated by the long-term administration of corticosteroids, hypertension, anemia, or disorders of the heart valves, CHF in lupus patients is managed with traditional remedies (e.g., digitalis, angiotensin-converting enzyme inhibitors, diuretics, β-blockers).

The Endocardium: Valvular Heart Disease

Materials such as cellular debris, proliferative cells, and immune complexes averaging 1 mm to 4 mm in diameter may form vegetations on cardiac valves in 1% to 5% of patients with SLE (Fig. 5.11). These sterile aggregates, termed "Libman-Sacks endocarditis," are especially observed in patients with antiphospholipid antibodies, as well as those who have been on long-term corticosteroid therapy. Morbidity ensues when these vegetations fleck off and travel to the brain, or become infected (especially after a dental procedure), becoming bacterial endocarditis. Identified by 2-D Doppler echocardiogram 30% of the

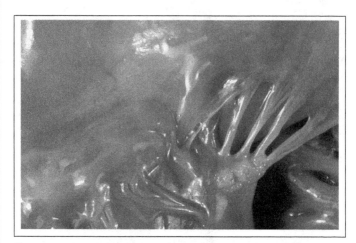

Figure 5.11 Libman-Sacks endocarditis. Note the valvular vegetation. ©1972–2004 American College of Rheumatology Clinical Slide Collection. Used with permission.

time, the lesions can be demonstrated by transesophageal echocardiography in 70% of patients.

Tricuspid regurgitation is a harbinger and symptom of pulmonary hypertension; mitral valve prolapse is slightly more frequent in SLE.

Hypertension

Patients with renal impairment, as well as those who have been on long-term corticosteroid therapy, are especially prone to blood pressure elevations. Hypertension is found in 25% to 30% of patients with SLE; it is also a contributing factor in accelerated atherogenesis (see next section).

Accelerated Atherogenesis

Coronary artery disease, hypertension, insulin resistance, metabolic syndrome, hyperhomocystinemia, and hyperlipidemia are more common in lupus patients, even in those for whom corticosteroids were never prescribed (Fig. 5.12). Several mechanisms may account for this, among them the presence of a recently described proinflammatory high-density lipoprotein (HDL) in 40% with SLE, the atherogenic effects of systemic inflammation, corticosteroids, and obesity related to lupus therapies. Recent work has concentrated on the dyslipidemia of lupus, oxidative stress, endothelial apoptosis, proinflammatory cytokines, adiponectin, leptin, and endothelial progenitor cells combined with traditional risk factors. Proactive screening for atherosclerotic disease (e.g., blood pressure monitoring, blood sugar and lipid testing, carotid duplex ultrasound, 2-D echocardiography, stress testing) with appropriate interventions (e.g., diet, exercise, smoking cessation, medication) can greatly diminish the morbidity and mortality of SLE.

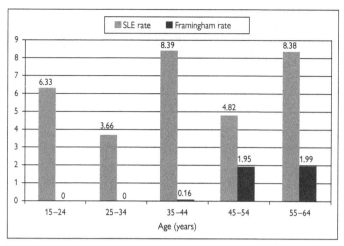

Figure 5.12 Incidence of myocardial infarction in 498 women with systemic lupus erythematosus. *Source*: Manzi S, Meilahn EN, Rairie JE, et al. Age-specific incidence rates of myocardial infarction and angina in women with systemic lupus erythematosus: comparison with the Framingham Study. *Am J Epidemiol.* 1997;145:408–415. Reprinted with permission, Oxford University Press, 1997.

The Nervous System

Lupus can involve the central, peripheral, and autonomic nervous systems. It produces myriad symptoms and signs that can be difficult to diagnose, to manage, and to differentiate from infection, psychological distress, or medication side effects. The 1982/1997 ACR criteria for nervous system involvement (seizures, psychosis) are obsolete. As a result, the ACR has delineated 19 different forms of nervous system lupus. Most lupus patients complain of at least some intermittent cognitive impairment; at least one of the 18 nervous system manifestations is noted in 30% of patients during the course of disease, and ongoing morbidity from such manifestations occurs in 10%[3] (Table 5.5).

Neurological Manifestations of Lupus

Memory impairment, confusion, and difficulty in articulating thoughts and remembering names or dates is termed *cognitive dysfunction*. "Lupus fog" is usually the result of a vascular-mediated process (e.g., bifrontal and bitemporal hyperperfusion on imaging studies) but can occur with headache, vasculitis, infection, and organic brain syndromes. *Headaches* are also usually autonomic/vascular in etiology but may be a manifestation of infection, medication, hypertension, vasculitis, or a cerebral bleed. *Seizures* result from inflammation, medication, fevers, or scar foci. *Altered consciousness* includes stupor, excessive sleepiness, or coma and is usually a consequence of active inflammation, medication, or infection. *Paralysis* or strokes can be sequelae of antiphospholipid antibodies or related to inflammation or atherosclerosis. *Movement disorders*

Table 5.5 Neuropsychiatric syndromes in systemic lupus erythematosus as defined by the American College of Rheumatology Research Committee

1. Central
   a. Aseptic meningitis
   b. Cardiovascular disease
   c. Demyelinating syndrome
   d. Headache
   e. Movement disorder
   f. Myelopathy
   g. Seizure disorders
   h. Acute confusional state
   i. Anxiety disorder
   j. Cognitive dysfunction
   k. Mood disorder
   l. Psychosis

2. Peripheral
   a. Guillain-Barré syndrome
   b. Autonomic neuropathy
   c. Mononeuropathy
   d. Myasthenia gravis
   e. Cranial neuropathy
   f. Plexopathy
   g. Polyneuropathy

include ataxia and chorea, resulting from infarction or inflammation of the cerebellum or basal ganglia. Corticosteroids, psychosocial distress, inflammation, and infection lead to *altered behavior* patterns. *Visual changes* may be produced by optic neuritis, pseudotumor cerebri, corticosteroids, cranial neuropathies, and other medications. Additional complaints include burning, numbness, and tingling from peripheral neuritis, cranial neuritis, dysautonomias, fibromyalgia, medication, or mechanical compression.

The Principal Lupus Syndromes of the Nervous System

Eighty percent of *CNS vasculitis* takes place in the first five years of disease. Seen in 10% of patients with SLE, it may be the initial presentation of the disorder. The typical patient experiences fevers, seizures, meningismus, and altered behavior patterns. If untreated, CNS vasculitis can progress to stupor, coma, status epilecticus, and death. Blood testing is unhelpful, brain imaging is nonspecific, and angiography has a less than 10% yield. Infection needs to be ruled out. Electroencephalograms and evoked responses are usually nonspecific and occasionally misleading. Spinal fluid evaluation is the gold standard: one-third of patients have pleocytosis, one-third have elevated protein, many have LE cells, and 80% demonstrate antineuronal antibodies. The most helpful test is the "multiple sclerosis panel"; the positive patient has oligoclonal bands and an increased IgG synthesis rate. Etiopathogenetic factors include perivascular or endothelial inflammation, vasculitis, hyalinization, infarction, hemorrhage, cytokine dysfunction, choroid plexus dysfunction, abnormal hypothalamic-pituitary-adrenal stress responses, and CNS tissue injury.

Lupus patients who develop sudden, nonpainful neurological deficits akin to a cerebrovascular accident (and these patients can be young) have *antiphospholipid syndrome*. Focal infarction is identified by neuroimaging and confirmed at physical examination. Nearly all patients will have an anticardiolipin antibody, prolonged clotting times, or a lupus anticoagulant. It is treated with anticoagulation. Other coagulopathies found in lupus and affecting the nervous system include *cryoglobulinemia*, *hyperviscosity*, or thromboembolic or bleeding complications from *thrombotic thrombocytopenic purpura* or *idiopathic thrombocytopenic purpura*. *Pseudotumor cerebri* (benign intracranial hypertension) is more common in SLE, as is *posterior reversible encephalopathy syndrome* (PRES), which manifests itself with severe hypertension and headache in patients who have received immune suppressive therapies.

Autonomic dysfunction in SLE involves vasomotor instability, which may produce migraine (*lupus headache*), or, conversely, transient cognitive impairment (*lupus fog*) resulting from excessive vasodilatation or vasoconstriction. Akin to "Raynaud's of the brain," dysautonomias are often mistaken or misinterpreted as lupus cerebritis, which they are not. Single-photon emission computed tomography, positron emission tomography, and functional magnetic resonance imaging demonstrate subtle flow abnormalities in the temporal-parietal, or watershed, regions. Extracranial manifestations of dysautonomia include palmar erythema, burning and tingling sensations, Raynaud's phenomenon, mitral valve prolapse, and livedo reticularis. Fibromyalgia needs to be ruled out. *Myelitis* may ensue from spinal cord inflammation or a coagulopathy that leads to paralysis or weakness. Normal spinal fluid findings with myelitis warrant anticoagulation, while corticosteroids are used if there is evidence for vasculitis.

CNS vasculitis, inflammation, or infarction heals but leaves scarring in the brain. Patients can have seizures or demonstrate cognitive dysfunction years after the incident episode. This is termed *organic brain syndrome*. It is managed with anticonvulsants, psychotropic drugs, and emotional support. Anti-inflammatory therapy in the absence of evidence for acute inflammation is contraindicated (Table 5.6).

The *peripheral nervous system* can become inflamed in 10% of persons with SLE. Manifesting itself as polyneuritis, cranial neuritis, myasthenia gravis, mononeuritis multiplex, or acute or chronic demyelinating inflammatory neuropathies (Guillain-Barré or Chronic inflammatory demyelinating polyneuropathy (CIDP)), peripheral inflammation can induce motor or sensory deficits identifiable on electromyography or nerve (especially sural) biopsy. Corticosteroids, immunosuppressive therapies, gabapentin derivatives, and, if necessary, intravenous immunoglobulin are the treatments of choice.

Head and Neck Manifestations, Including Sjögren's Syndrome

The Eye

Discoid lesions around the eye are not uncommon. Conjunctivitis and episcleritis are more frequently noted in SLE. Uveitis is statistically associated with lupus

Table 5.6 Major central nervous system (CNS) syndromes and their management

Syndrome	Prevalence in lupus (%)	Treatment
Cerebral vasculitis	10	High-dose IV steroids, immunosuppressants
Antiphospholipid syndrome	5 to 10	Platelet inhibition, anticoagulants with brain clots
Lupus headache	15	Migraine therapy, steroids
Cognitive dysfunction	50	Antimalarials, psychotropics, biofeedback counseling, cognitive-behavioral therapy
Fibromyalgia	10 to 20	Nonsteroidals, counseling, psychotropics, physical therapy
CNS infection	1	Antibiotics
Cryoglobulinemia or hyperviscosity	1	Steroids, apheresis, immunosuppressants
Bleed due to low platelets	2	Steroids, apheresis, chemotherapy, factor replacement, transfusion

but seen in only 1% to 2% of patients. Corticosteroid therapy is the source of most cataracts and glaucoma diagnosed in lupus patients. Antimalarial therapies can produce retinal changes in 3% of patients taking hydroxychloroquine and 10% of patients taking chloroquine for 10 years. Between 1% and 2% of patients with SLE develop retinal vasculitis or optic neuritis (Fig. 5.13). Antiphospholipid antibody–mediated clots in the retina need to be considered in the differential diagnosis.

The Ear, Nose, and Throat

One lupus patient in 500 develops autoimmune vestibulitis, which presents with a sudden onset of hearing deficits that are steroid-responsive. Lupus chondritis inflames the ear cartilage and is rapidly responsive to moderate-dose corticosteroids. Mucocutaneous lesions are discussed in an earlier section of this chapter. A hoarse voice is noted when the synovially lined cricoarytenoid joint is inflamed. Patients with SLE who undergo dental work should receive routine antibiotic prophylaxis if they are immune-suppressed or have additional risk factors (e.g., Libman-Sacks endocarditis).

Periodontal disease is more common in lupus patients who also have Sjögren's and scleroderma overlaps.

Sjögren's Syndrome

Characterized by dry eyes and dry mouth (keratoconjunctivitis sicca), Sjögren's is diagnosed when these manifestations are related to an immunological dysfunction of the exocrine (lacrimal and salivary) glands. Secondary Sjögren's is

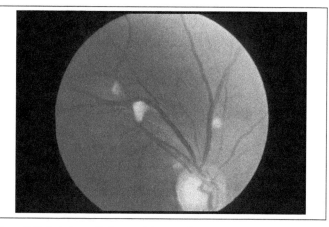

Figure 5.13 Retinal vasculitis in systemic lupus erythematosus. ©1972–2004 American College of Rheumatology Clinical Slide Collection. Used with permission.

found in 10% to 20% of persons with SLE and is diagnosed by a combination of factors, including parotid enlargement; Lissimine green or Rose-Bengal staining or Schirmer testing of the cornea; positive anti-SSA (Ro) antibodies; and evidence for a dry mouth by lip biopsy, salivary imaging, or flow tests. Dry lungs (bronchitis sicca), vaginal dryness, and renal tubular acidosis are associated features. Sjögren's-specific remedies, in addition to lupus therapies, include topical replacement of lubrication, sialogogues, cyclosporine eye drops, and pilocarpine. These are summarized in Table 5.7.

Endocrinopathies

Autoimmune thyroiditis, type 1 diabetes, autoimmune adrenalitis, premenstrual disease flares, and elevated prolactin levels have increased prevalence in SLE.

Gastrointestinal Manifestations

The gastrointestinal tract is rarely directly involved in SLE. Dysphagia and esophageal motility disorders are seen in scleroderma and inflammatory myositis overlaps. Comorbidities such as GERD or gastritis (due to corticosteroids

Table 5.7 Clinical features of Sjögren's syndrome

COMMON: Dry eyes (keratoconjunctivitis sicca), dry mouth (xerostomia), arthralgias

FOUND IN 10%–50% WITH SJOGREN'S: Parotid gland enlargement, dry cough (bronchitis sicca), vaginal dryness, atrophic gastritis, hypothyroidism

FOUND IN <10% OF PATIENTS: Peripheral nerve disease, pancreatitis, renal tubular acidosis, interstitial lung disease, lymphoma

or nonsteroidal therapies), nausea or diarrhea (due to steroids, nonsteroidals, antimalarials, or immune suppressives), and peptic ulcer disease (due to medication) are prevalent in lupus. SLE is statistically associated with ulcerative colitis, biliary cirrhosis, celiac disease, autoimmune hepatitis, and autoimmune pancreatitis. Direct lupus involvement of the gastrointestinal tract manifests as ascites (especially with nephrosis—seen at some point in 10%), protein-losing enteropathy (almost always limited to children and adolescents), and pancreatitis. The latter results from medications (e.g., diuretics, azathioprine, corticosteroids), biliary cirrhosis, usual causes of pancreatitis (e.g., gallstones, alcohol abuse), or frank pancreatic vasculitis (found in 1% of those with SLE). Mesenteric vasculitis with ensuing infarction is a life-threatening complication of SLE noted in 1% to 2% with the disease. An antiphospholipid-mediated process should first be ruled out, and aggressive high-dose corticosteroids should be administered, along with close surgical coordination.

Low-level liver enzyme abnormalities may ensue from nonsteroidal anti-inflammatory drugs, salicylates, methotrexate, and fatty livers exacerbated by corticosteroid therapy. Usually, no treatment is necessary. Hepatitis due to SLE is diagnosed once viral etiologies are ruled out. Autoimmune hepatitis can coexist with or be part of lupus and responds to corticosteroid and immunosuppressive regimens (e.g., azathioprine, 6mercaptopurine). Budd-Chiari syndrome is associated with antiphospholipid antibodies.

Lupus in the Kidneys and Urinary Tract

Pathophysiology

Classic chronic immune complex glomerulonephritis, as defined in experimental models, is strikingly similar to what is seen in human SLE. Autoantibodies bind to nonglomerular autoantigens, intrinsic glomerular antigens, and preformed circulating immune complexes, which are deposited in the glomerulus. Nucleosomes in the form of DNA bound to histone have an affinity for anionic components of the glomerular basement membrane such as heparan sulfate, which bind to negatively charged cell surfaces or matrix components of the glomerulus in the course of filtration. Nucleosomal antigen interacts with circulating autoantibody, leading to the formation of immune complexes in situ. This results in activation of the complement cascade, procoagulant factors, monocyte and neutrophil infiltration, release of proteolytic enzymes, elaboration of various cytokines and adhesion molecules, and consequent glomerular and vascular damage. Hypertension further accelerates this.

Lupus Nephritis

Thirty percent of individuals with SLE have some form of renal involvement; in half of these cases, it mandates organ-specific therapy. Unless one has nephrosis or is uremic, lupus nephritis is usually asymptomatic. It may be present in concert with multisystem complaints or found incidentally via routine urinalysis. The report of urinary casts (hyaline or granular) and/or hematuria along with proteinuria should lead one to suspect renal involvement. Most lupus specialists now agree that a renal biopsy is the gold standard that guides the diagnosis and treatment of lupus. First, it usually rules out diabetes, hypertension, other forms of vasculitis, amyloidosis, hepatitis, and lymphoma, among other conditions that can mimic lupus nephritis. The advent of interventional radiology and ultrasonography has made the biopsy procedure much safer. The World Health Organization's 1982 histopathological classifications have given way to the 2004 International Society of Nephrology and Renal Pathology Society (ISN/RPS) revisions, which take into account damage and activity indices evolved by the National Institutes of Health in the mid-1980s.[4] (See Tables 5.8 and 5.9 and Figs. 5.14 through 5.17.) Whereas nil disease (Class I) and mesangial disease (Class II) have excellent prognoses, patients with proliferative or membranous nephritis have a 50% and 30% risk of evolving end-stage renal disease within 10 years, respectively. Lupus nephritis is associated with high morbidity and mortality. In addition to renal failure, the potential for hypertension, hyperlipidemia, Cushing's disease, electrolyte disorders, insulin resistance, and nephrotic syndrome mandates extra vigilance. Patients should be proactively screened and treated for these complications. Diet, angiotensin-converting enzyme inhibitors, weight control, exercise, and specific attention to medication adherence are important in the management of lupus nephritis. Renal lupus is monitored by C3 complement and anti-DNA (usually abnormal with proliferative nephritis but normal in burnt-out disease or membranous nephritis), serum albumin levels, monitoring of vital signs, 24-hour urinary protein or protein-to-creatinine determinations, glomerular filtration rate calculations, and blood chemistry panels. Individuals with antiphospholipid antibodies and nephritis often demonstrate pathological evidence for microthrombi and atheroembolic events; renal vein thrombosis is associated with these antibodies and membranous nephritis. Sjögren's patients may have coexisting renal tubular acidosis and interstitial disease.

Table 5.8 Histopathological directed treatment approaches for lupus nephritis

Biopsy class	Name	10-year dialysis risk (%)	Treatment
I	Nil	<1	None
II	Mesangial	10	20 mg prednisone × 3 months
III•	Focal proliferative	50	Steroids, immunosuppressants
IV•	Diffuse proliferative	50 to 75	Steroids, immunosuppressants
V•	Membranous	30	Steroids, immunosuppressants
VI	Glomerulosclerosis	High	None

• Steroid regimen: 1 mg/kg/day prednisone equivalent for 6 weeks followed by 10% week tapering to 10 mg/day maintenance for 2 years

• Immunosuppressive regimen: Cyclophosphamide 750 mg/m² × 6 dose initiation with q 3 month dosing for 2 years, and/or mycophenolate mofetil 2 to 3 g/day OR azathioprine 150 mg/day AND/OR Rituximab 1 g given in divided doses 2 weeks apart q 6 months.

Table 5.9 International Society of Nephrology and Renal Pathology Society (ISN/RPS) classification of lupus nephritis (2004)

Class I	Minimal mesangial: normal glomeruli by light microscopy (LM), mesangial immune deposits by immunofluorescence
Class II	Mesangial proliferative: mesangial hypercellularity or matrix expansion by LM with mesangial immune deposits
Class III	Focal proliferative: focal, segmental, and/or global endo- and/or extra-capillary involvement of <50% of glomeruli, with or without mesangial alterations
	III (A): purely active lesions
	III (A/C): active and chronic lesions
	III (C): Chronic inactive with scarring
Class IV	Diffuse proliferative: same as Class III but involving >50% of glomeruli
	IV-S (A) or IV-G (A): purely active, diffuse segmental or global proliferative
	IV-S (A/C) or IV-G (A/C): above with active and chronic lesions
	IV-S (C) or IV-G (C): inactive with scarring
Class V	Membranous: global or segmental subepithelial immune deposits with or without mesangial alteration
Class VI	Advanced sclerosing: >90% of glomeruli sclerosed with no activity

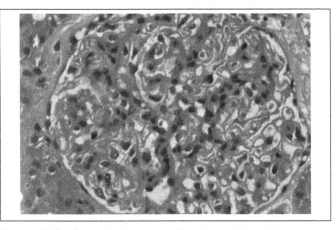

Figure 5.14 Class II mesangial disease. *Source*: Wallace DJ, Hahn BH. *Dubois' Lupus Erythematosus*, 7th ed. Philadelphia, PA: Lippincott Williams & Wilkins; 2007. Reprinted with permission.

Lupus Cystitis and Bladder Disturbances

Urinary tract infections are extremely common in young women with SLE. Sulfa antibiotics used by practitioners to manage these may lead to a disease flare or sun sensitization and should be carefully prescribed, or avoided. Hemorrhagic cystitis can be a manifestation of active lupus or cyclophosphamide therapy.

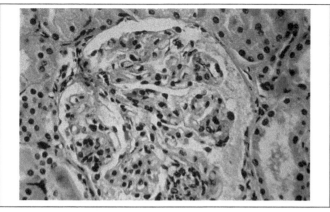

Figure 5.15 Class III focal proliferative nephritis. ©1972–2004 American College of Rheumatology Clinical Slide Collection. Used with permission.

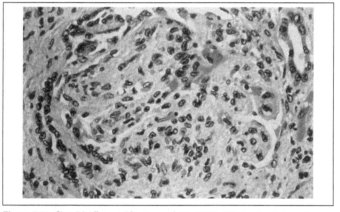

Figure 5.16 Class IV diffuse proliferative nephritis. ©1972–2004 American College of Rheumatology Clinical Slide Collection. Used with permission.

The Hemic-Lymphatic System

Anemias

Over 80% of lupus patients are anemic at some point in time. Most have anemia as a chronic disease. Young women with heavy menses lose iron as well. Lupus medications ranging from nonsteroidal anti-inflammatory agents to immunosuppressive regimens further contribute to the anemia cauldron. Renal impairment is an additional anemogenic contributor. Autoimmune disease is associated with atrophic gastritis with resulting vitamin B_{12} deficiency. The management of anemia in lupus depends on its source.[9]

Autoimmune hemolytic anemia (AIHA) occurs in up to 10% of individuals with SLE. AIHA is suspected when lupus patients are anemic and have elevated

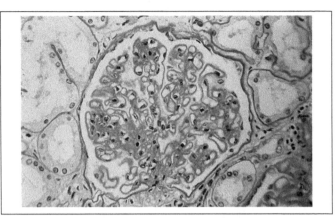

Figure 5.17 Class V membranous nephritis. ©1972–2004 American College of Rheumatology Clinical Slide Collection. Used with permission.

serum lactate dehydrogenase (LDH) and reticulocyte counts, decreased serum haptoglobin, or a positive Coombs' direct test, and diagnosis is confirmed when the peripheral blood smear is viewed (see Table 5.10).

Leukopenia, Leukocytosis, and Adenopathy

Leukopenia is seen in almost all lupus patients at some time. A consequence of antilymphocyte antibodies, viral infection, medication, or bone marrow suppression, this benign finding is considered to be a marker of disease activity and very rarely mandates a specific intervention. Leukocytosis with lymphopenia results from corticosteroid therapy. Granulocytopenia is rare in SLE and warrants consideration of other diagnoses (e.g., Felty's syndrome).

Adenopathy and reactive lymphadenitis are markers of active disease and are found in half of all lupus patients at some point in the disease course. Sometimes the glands are so large (Kikuchi's syndrome) that a biopsy may be performed to rule out other conditions. Ten percent of lupus patients have an enlarged spleen on CT of the abdomen.

Table 5.10 Sources of anemia in SLE
1. Anemia of chronic disease
2. Iron deficiency
3. Folic acid or B_{12} deficiency
4. Bone marrow suppression
5. Drugs (e.g., NSAIDs, immune suppressives)
6. Sickle-cell anemia
7. Renal impairment
8. Immune anemias (e.g., hemolytic, thrombotic thrombocytopenic purpura)
9. Heavy menses

Platelet Defects, Including Idiopathic Thrombocytopenic Purpura and Thrombotic Thrombocytopenic Purpura

Qualitative platelet defects are noted in a few lupus patients not taking any medication, but are primarily induced by aspirin, nonsteroidal drugs, and corticosteroids. Some patients manifest purpura or ecchymoses. Prolonged clotting times are found with the lupus anticoagulant and antiphospholipid antibodies.

Low platelet counts are observed in lupus patients taking immunosuppressive medication and in those with infections, idiopathic thrombocytopenic purpura (ITP), and thrombotic thrombocytopenic purpura (TTP). ITP is a common immune thrombocytopenia in that 20% with SLE have antiplatelet antibodies, and in 20% of these patients, platelet counts drop below 100,000/mm^3. Most lupus specialists treat thrombocytopenia when counts decrease to 60,000/mm^3 or fewer.

TTP is a rare, life-threatening complication of SLE consisting of a pentad of fever, nephritis, hemolysis, renal impairment, and neurological compromise that mimics or can be brought on by an infection. The diagnosis is confirmed by assessing the functional activity of a disintegrin and metalloproteinase with a thrombospondin type 1 motif, member 13 (ADAMTS13) (a von Willebrand factor protease) and viewing the peripheral blood smear.

References

1. Wallace DJ, Hahn BH. Sections IV and V: The skin in lupus and clinical aspects of lupus. In: DJ Wallace and BH Hahn, eds. *Dubois' Lupus Erythematosus*. 7th ed. Philadelphia, PA: Lippincott Williams & Wilkins; 2007:551–1130.

2. Patel P, Werth V. Cutaneous lupus erythematosus: a review. *Dermatol Clin.* 2002;20:373–385.

3. Hanly JG. ACR classification criteria for systemic lupus erythematosus: limitations and revisions to neuropsychiatric variables. *Lupus*. 2004;13:861–864.

4. Weening JJ, D'Agati VD, Schwartz MM, et al. The classification of glomerulonephritis in systemic lupus erythematosus revisited. *J Am Soc Nephrol.* 2004;15:241–250.

5. van Vugt R, Derksen R, Kater L, et al. Deforming arthropathy or lupus and rhupus hands in patients with systemic lupus erythematosus. *Ann Rheum Dis.* 1998;57:540–544.

6. McMahon M, Skaggs B, Grossman J. Pathogenesis and treatment of atherosclerosis in lupus. In: DJ Wallace and BH Hahn, eds. *Dubois' Lupus Erythematosus and Related Syndromes*. 8th ed. Philadelphia, PA: Elsevier; 2013:341–351.

7. Keane MP, Lynch JP. Pleuropulmonary manifestations of systemic lupus erythematosus. *Thorax*. 2000;55:159–166.

8. Karpouzis GA. Hematologic and lymphoid abnormalities in SLE. In: DJ Wallace and BH Hahn, eds. *Dubois' Lupus Erythematosus and Related Syndromes*. 8th edition. Philadelphia, PA: Elsevier; 2013:426–437.

Chapter 6

Laboratory and Imaging Abnormalities

Routine Testing in General Medical Offices

A typical primary care physician's clinical laboratory and imaging center allows him or her to successfully diagnose, stage, and monitor response to therapy in lupus patients. The complete blood count screens for anemia, autoimmune hemolytic anemia, leucopenia, lymphopenia, leukocytosis, and thrombocytopenias. A comprehensive metabolic panel, along with lipid and thyroid testing, evaluates liver, renal, and metabolic functions. A routine urinalysis shows sediment, casts, or protein excretion in individuals with renal involvement. Muscle enzymes are elevated with myositis. The partial thromboplastin time is prolonged in many patients with the lupus anticoagulant. Acute-phase reactants such as erythrocyte sedimentation rate and C-reactive protein are elevated with active disease. Chest radiographs reveal pleural effusions, pleural scarring, and interstitial or alveolar changes, while electrocardiograms may suggest pericarditis or myocarditis as well as screen for infarction, strain patterns, or arrhythmias. Joint imaging screens for erosions, calcinosis, and avascular necrosis.[1]

Table 6.1 provides a summary of the levels and type of testing useful in managing lupus patients.[2]

Useful, Readily Available, Community-Based Testing

Lupus practitioners may order readily available testing outside of their clinic or office that may be useful in specific settings. Examples include a 2-D echocardiogram to screen for pulmonary hypertension or pericardial effusion, electromyography with nerve conduction velocities to confirm the presence of myositis or neuropathies, electroencephalography for seizures, computed tomography (CT) scans to confirm or evaluate splenomegaly and interstitial lung disease, and magnetic resonance imaging for avascular necrosis or cerebritis, among others (Table 6.1).

Complement

The complement system comprises more than 30 plasma- and membrane-bound proteins designed to protect against invading pathogens.

Table 6.1 Summary of useful tests used in systemic lupus erythematosus

Level 1: Routine screening for all patients (total cost <$500)• Complete blood count
- Comprehensive metabolic profile
- Urinalysis
- Muscle enzymes (e.g., creatine phosphokinase)
- Acute-phase reactants (e.g., C-reactive protein or sedimentation rate)
- Chest radiograph
- Electrocardiogram
- Antinuclear antibody
- C3 or C4 complement
- Anti-dsDNA

Level 2: Readily available, inexpensive testing for selected patients
- Partial thromboplastin time
- 2-D echocardiography
- Hand or feet radiographs
- Rheumatoid factor
- Bone densitometry

Level 3: Reflex panel testing to characterize nature of lupus involvement
- Anti-extractable nuclear antigen panel (anti-Sm, -RNP, -SSA, -SSB)
- Antiphospholipid panel (syphilis serology, lupus anticoagulant, anticardiolipin)

Level 4: Specialized testing limited to selected clinical circumstances
- Computed tomography or magnetic resonance imaging
- Electrical studies (e.g., electroencephalography, electromyography)
- Niche serologies (e.g., antihistone, chromatin, neuronal, ribosomal P)
- Bone scan

Most exist in the plasma as functionally inactive proproteins until appropriate events trigger their activation. Classical and alternative pathways involve C1–C4, among other proteins, which converge into a membrane attack complex consisting of C5b–C9. A hereditary deficiency of C1, C2, or C4 has been associated with the development of SLE (relevant in less than 1% of patients). In systemic lupus erythematosus patients, decreased serum levels of C3 and C4 components are usually associated with inflammation and correlate with disease activity.

Serological Evaluations

The antinuclear antibody (ANA) is considered the gold standard for identifying SLE. Positive in 96% of those with the disease, it has very poor specificity and can be present in up to 10% of a healthy population, and may be found in patients with other autoimmune conditions (Table 6.2).[3] ANA-negative lupus is usually seen in patients with chronic cutaneous disease or antiphospholipid syndrome or in individuals who have had long-term corticosteroid or immunosuppressive therapy, during which a positive ANA becomes negative. Titers are of little value, but higher numbers are associated with autoimmune disorders.

Table 6.2 Hypercoagulability in SLE: A Venn diagram of overlapping features.
Prevalence of ANA in the US
Cross-sectional analysis of 4754 NHANES individuals
13.8% older than 12 years of age were positive
Prevalence higher among
• African Americans
• Females
• Older individuals
32 million people in the US have elevated ANAs, fewer than 1 million have lupus, but 98%
Satoh M. *Arthritis Rheum*. 2012;64:2319–2327. Kavanaugh A, et al. *Arch Pathol Lab Med*. 2000;124(1):71–81.

A homogeneous or rimmed pattern on immune fluorescence is suggestive of lupus, whereas speckled patterns are nonspecific, and nucleolar or centromere staining suggests a scleroderma component.

Most laboratories have a "reflex panel," whereby additional serologies are performed if the antinuclear antibody is positive.[4] Over 140 autoantibodies have been identified in rheumatic diseases. Those clinically relevant to SLE are reviewed in this section. Antibodies to nuclear components of the cell include anti-DNA, antihistone, antichromatin, and antibodies to extractable nuclear antigens (ENAs) (e.g., anti-Sm/RNP). Antibodies to double-stranded DNA are present in half of those with lupus; positively charged antibodies can directly damage tissue and are especially important in nephritis. If measured by a Farr or enzyme-linked immunosorbent assay (ELISA), anti-DNA levels are used to follow the patient's response to therapy. Antihistone antibodies are present in drug-induced lupus and a small percentage of those with rheumatoid arthritis. These structural proteins are responsible for the LE cell phenomenon. Antichromatin antibodies appear phylogenetically before anti-DNA and are usually fairly specific for the presence of SLE but are of little clinical significance. The anti-Sm (or Smith) antibody is named after the patient in whom it was first reported, and it interferes with one's ability to transcribe RNA from DNA. It is seen in 20% of those with SLE but less than 1% of healthy individuals. Following its levels is of no clinical value. Antibodies to ribonucleoprotein are seen in low titers in SLE patients and in higher titers in those with mixed connective tissue disease. By definition, the diagnosis of MCTD is not possible without anti-RNP. This antibody interferes with the ability of RNA to bind in the cytoplasm of cells. Clinically, individuals with moderate to high titers of anti-RNP have puffy hands, Raynaud's phenomenon, and an increased prevalence of pulmonary hypertension.

The principal antibodies to cytoplasmic components include antibodies to Ro and La (also known as the Sjögren's antibodies, SS-A and SS-B). Anti-Ro is found in the majority of patients with primary Sjögren's syndrome and approximately 20% to 30% of those with SLE. It interferes with the cell's ability to process RNA and is clinically associated with increased photosensitivity and subacute cutaneous lupus. Anti-Ro has the ability to cross the placenta, and its

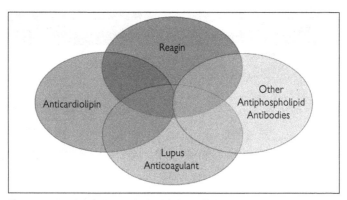

Figure 6.1 Antiphospholipid antibodies In 1/3 with SLE, 1/3 of whom have APS.

52-kDa protein can induce a transient rash in newborns (known as *neonatal lupus*) or congenital heart block. Anti-Ro is 50% more common than anti-La, and the latter may mitigate some of the injury associated with the former. La functions as a way station on the road to where RNA transcripts are carried from the nucleus to the cytoplasm. Antibodies to ribosomal P are seen in 20% of individuals with SLE. Its levels are not important in lupus treatment, but they do clinically correlate with liver injury, depression, and psychosis. Antibodies to phospholipids in cell membranes are features of the antiphospholipid syndrome[5,6] (see Fig. 6.1).

Antibodies to cellular components noted in lupus include antierythrocyte, antilymphocyte, antiplatelet, antineutrophil (antineutrophil cytoplasmic antibodies [ANCA]), and antineuronal antibodies. These are markers of damage to these cells and are infrequently useful in a clinical setting. Additionally, antibodies form against circulating antigens. Rheumatoid factor is reported in 30% with SLE and is nonspecific, although joint inflammation is more common in these patients. Last, circulating immune complexes can vary according to charge, avidity, size, antigen excess, or antibody excess, and are rarely followed. Their levels are increased in active lupus as well as in a variety of infections (see Table 6.3).

Table 6.3 Important autoantibodies and antibodies in lupus				
Autoantibody	**Antibody to:**	**% in SLE**	**% in normals**	**Lupus specificity**
Antinuclear	Nucleus	98	5 to 10	Fair
Anti-dsDNA	Nucleus	50	<1	Excellent
Antihistone	Nucleus	50	1 to 3	Fair
Anti-Sm	Nucleus	25	<1	Excellent
Anti-RNP	Nucleus	25	<1	Fair
APL	Membrane	33	5	Fair

(continued)

Table 6.3 (Continued)				
Autoantibody	Antibody to:	% in SLE	% in normals	Lupus specificity
Anti-Ro (SSA)	Cytoplasm	30	<1	Fair
Anti-La (SSB)	Cytoplasm	15	<1	Fair
Anti-ribosomal P	Cytoplasm	20	<1	Good
Antierythrocyte	Red cells	15 to 30	<1	Fair
ANCA	White cells	20	<1	Poor
Antilymphocyte	White cells	Most	20	Poor
Antiplatelet	Platelets	15 to 30	<5	Poor
Antineuronal	Nerve cells	20	<1	Good
Rheumatoid factor	Ag-Ab	30	5 to 10	Poor
Immune complexes	Ag-Ab	Most	Varies	Poor
Anti-CCP	Ag-Ab	5	<1	Poor

Key: APL, antiphospholipid antibody; RNP, ribonucleoprotein; ANCA, antineutrophil cytoplasmic antibody; CCP, cyclic citrullinated peptide. Source: Wallace DJ. The Lupus Book, 5th ed. New York: Oxford University Press; 2012. Used with permission.

References

1. Sheldon J. Laboratory testing in autoimmune rheumatic diseases. Best Pract Res Clin Rheumatol. 2004;18:249–269.

2. Wallace DJ, Schwartz E, Lin H-C, Peter JB. The "rule-out lupus" rheumatology consultation: clinical outcomes and perspectives. J Clin Rheumatol. 1995;1:158–164.

3. Kurien BT, Scofield RH. Autoantibody testing in the diagnosis of systemic lupus erythematosus. Scand J Immunol. 2006;64:227–235.

4. Sherer Y, Gorstem A, Fritzler MJ, Shoenfeld Y. Autoantibody explosion in systemic lupus: more than 100 different autoantibodies found in SLE patients. Semin Arthritis Rheum. 2004;34:501–537.

5. Satoh M, Chan EK, Ho LA. Prevalence and sociodemographic correlates of anti-nuclear antibodies in the United States. Arthritis Rheum. 2012;64:2319–2327.

6. Kavanaugh A, Romar R, Reveille J, et al. Guidelines for clinical use of the antinuclear tests for specific autoantibodies and nuclear antigens. Arch Pathol Lab Med. 2000;124:71–81.

Chapter 7

Differential Diagnosis and Disease Associations

Lupus has many similarities to the "great mimicker," as Sir William Osler termed syphilis. It can present with symptoms, signs, and laboratory abnormalities affecting every organ system in the body. Twenty percent of patients with one autoimmune disease (including lupus) have a second autoimmune disorder. As a result, there is often a great degree of confusion when lupus is part of the differential diagnosis. This chapter addresses these issues.[1]

Rheumatoid Arthritis

Rheumatoid arthritis (RA) is an inflammatory disorder primarily affecting the synovium. Twice as prevalent as SLE, it most often presents with bilateral, symmetrical aching and stiffness along with swelling primarily of the small joints of the hands and feet. The wrists, knees, hips, and shoulders are also involved. RA has several features that tend to differentiate it from lupus: erosive joint disease on imaging studies, antibodies to cyclic citrullinated peptide (CCP), rheumatoid nodules, and a greater degree of synovitis. Constitutional symptoms and signs of fevers and fatigue are common. Extra-articular findings are observed in only 15% of persons with RA, and include rheumatoid lung, serositis, and cutaneous vasculitis; 70% are rheumatoid-factor positive, as opposed to 30% with SLE, but 50% with RA have antinuclear antibodies. During the first year of symptoms, RA and SLE can be impossible to tell apart. Lupus is usually suspected if cutaneous or organ-threatening disease is evident. Approximately 1% to 5% of persons with RA also meet the American College of Rheumatology (ACR) criteria for SLE and are said to have "rhupus." Although the treatments of the two disorders overlap to some extent, sulfasalazine has no place in the treatment of lupus, and anti–tumor necrosis factor blockers are less useful.[2]

Scleroderma

Patients with scleroderma can display sclerodactyly, Raynaud's phenomenon, calcinosis, gastrointestinal dysmotility, telangiectasias, generalized skin tightening, pulmonary hypertension, interstitial lung disease, myocardial fibrosis, and digital acral osteolysis, among other features. Raynaud's phenomenon is found in 30% of persons with SLE, as opposed to 90% with scleroderma; the additional above-listed features are found in less than 10% with lupus. SLE patients with scleroderma manifestations usually have mixed connective tissue disease or overlap syndrome. Autoantibodies found in scleroderma (e.g., anticentromere antibody, anti-SCL antibody) occur in less than 5% of persons with lupus. Pure lupus rarely heals its inflammation with the exuberant fibrosis found in scleroderma, and endothelial cell dysfunction and intimal hyperplasia with vascular compromise are also uncommon in SLE.

Inflammatory Myositis

Although MCTD and overlap syndrome patients with concurrent SLE may have myositis, and though the histology of a dermatomyositis rash is identical to that of lupus, there are some important differences. Creatine phosphokinase (CK) determinations rarely exceed 1000 units in lupus, Gottron's papules are absent, and heliotrope distribution rashes are not seen in SLE. Proximal weakness due to myositis is not found. The degree of calcinosis is much less than that in juvenile dermatomyositis, and malignancies are much more frequent in older individuals with dermatomyositis. Myositis antibodies (e.g., anti-Jo, anti-PM-1) are not noted in lupus.

The Vasculidites

Lupus affects the small and medium-sized arterioles, as do certain forms of vasculitis such as microscopic polyangiitis and polyarteritis nodosa. Antinuclear cytoplasmic antibodies (ANCA) may be present in up to 20% of persons with SLE, but without the proteinase-3 or myeloperoxidase staining found with Wegener's granulomatosis or microscopic polyangiitis. Eosinophilia is common in polyarteritis but rare in lupus. Polymyalgia rheumatica mimics early lupus in older patients, but these individuals usually only have constitutional or musculoskeletal manifestations. Unlike Takayasu arteritis or temporal arteritis, large vessels are involved in less than 1% of lupus patients. Granulomatous responses are a feature of Wegener's granulomatosis, Churg-Strauss syndrome, and sarcoidosis, but not lupus. In older patients, polymyalgia rheumatica can be difficult to differentiate from SLE, but it tends to limit itself to the musculoskeletal system.

Seronegative Spondyloarthropathies, Inflammatory Bowel Disease, and Behçet's

Ankylosing spondylitis, reactive arthritis, and psoriatic arthritis coexist with lupus at the same or lower prevalence than in the general population due to male predominance. Occasionally, women with a low-titer antinuclear antibody and inflammatory arthritis or inflammatory bowel disease are misdiagnosed as having SLE. This family of diseases should be suspected when the HLA-B27 is positive. Anti-DNA, anticardiolipin, and antinuclear antibodies can develop from treatment with tumor necrosis factor inhibitors, used to manage ulcerative colitis or Crohn's disease, as a "drug-induced lupus." Some consider Behçet's to fall into the seronegative spondyloarthropathy category. Young women with a low-titer antinuclear antibody, mucocutaneous lesions, and central nervous system vasculitis can be mislabeled as having lupus. Behçet's patients may have a positive pathergy test, absence of autoantibodies, and erythema nodosum not usually seen with lupus, as well as prominent uveitis or cerebellar abnormalities, and they are not responsive to antimalarials.

Sarcoidosis

Sarcoid and SLE patients share a similar demographic: young African American females. Sarcoidosis is differentiated from SLE by hilar changes on chest radiographs, elevated angiotensin-converting enzyme blood testing, and the presence of non-caseating granulomas.

Infections

Infections can activate a predisposition to lupus, and lupus patients are especially susceptible to infections. Fevers (especially in those on steroids or immunosuppressives) should raise the suspicion of an underlying infectious process, opportunistic or otherwise. Certain microbial infections are associated with the production of antinuclear antibody. Early lupus can be confused with parvovirus, Epstein-Barr, cytomegalovirus, hepatitis, and other related conditions. Human immunodeficiency virus has a negative correlation with SLE (they are immunological opposites), but some lupus patients have false-positive blood testing for the virus. Lyme disease patients may have a false-positive syphilis serology (it is a spirochete), and symptoms may be misread as lupus. Tuberculosis and leprosy attack the joints and produce lupus-like skin lesions, but associated granulomas are not found in SLE. Herpes zoster is extremely common in immunosuppressed patients.

Fibromyalgia

Fibromyalgia (FM) is a central sensitization syndrome associated with prominent complaints of fatigue, aching, alteration in sleep architecture, and tender points. Other central sensitization syndromes include functional bowel disorders, irritable bladder, chronic pelvic pain, chronic fatigue syndrome, and tension headache. Corticosteroid dose change or withdrawal and psychosocial stressors can cause or aggravate FM. Hence, 20% to 30% of persons with SLE also fulfill the ACR criteria for FM at some point in the course of their disease. Some FM patients with nonspecific constitutional symptoms and a low-titer antinuclear antibody are difficult to differentiate from those with SLE. This author requires evidence for inflammation (e.g., elevation of sedimentation rate, C-reactive protein, low C3 complement), urinary sediment, a positive serology other than antinuclear antibody, significant cytopenias, or tissue biopsy demonstrating vasculitis before initiating any anti-inflammatory regimen other than nonsteroidal anti-inflammatory drugs.

Table 7.1 The differential diagnosis of systemic lupus erythematosus

Autoimmune disorders
- Rheumatoid arthritis
- Scleroderma
- Inflammatory myositis
- Vasculitis
- Seronegative spondyloarthropathies
- Inflammatory bowel disorders
- Behçet's
- Sarcoidosis
- Palindromic rheumatism
- Sjögren's syndrome
- Polymyalgia rheumatica
- Autoimmune thyroiditis
- Undifferentiated connective tissue disease

Infections (especially Epstein-Barr, chronic Lyme, tuberculosis)

Fibromyalgia

Allergies

Neurological disorders (e.g., myasthenia gravis, multiple sclerosis)

Malignancy (especially lymphoproliferative disorders)

Psychiatric disorders (e.g., bipolar illness, malnutrition, substance abuse)

Endocrine/Hormonal (e.g., hypothyroidism)

Additional Considerations

Hormonal imbalances (especially Hashimoto's thyroiditis with an elevated level of thyroid-stimulating hormone), neurological disorders, carcinoma, pregnancy, and psychiatric disorders can be misdiagnosed as SLE.[3] Important differential considerations are listed in Table 7.1.[4]

References

1. Rooney J. Systemic lupus erythematosus: unmasking a great imitator. *Nursing.* 2005;35:54–60.

2. Shmerling RH. Diagnostic tests for rheumatic disease: clinical utility revisited. *South Med J.* 2005;98:704–713.

3. Maddison PJ. Is it SLE? *Best Prac Res Clin Rheumatol.* 2002;16:167–180.

4. Jolly M, Francis S, Sequiera W. Differential diagnosis and disease associations, in DJ Wallace and BH Hahn, eds. *Dubois' Lupus Erythematosus and Related Disorders,* 8th ed. Philadelphia, PA: Elsevier; 2013:541–554.

Chapter 8

Important Subsets and Special Considerations

Lupus Through the Ages: Neonatal, Childhood, Adolescence, and Elderly

When antibodies to Ro (SSA) cross the placenta, they infrequently settle in fetal tissue. Anti-SSB and anti-RNP may do this as well. *Neonatal lupus* occurs when the infant is born with a discoid or subacute cutaneous rash that disappears within weeks, often without treatment[1] (Fig. 8.1). This occurs in 7% of infants born to anti-Ro-positive mothers. Two percent of the time, this antibody settles in other tissues. Of those with pathology, 54% have varying degrees of myocardial dysfunction, and 7% have hepatic, hematological, or neurological complications. Pregnant mothers with anti-Ro should undergo serial fetal echocardiograms between weeks 18 and 24; dexamethasone or intravenous immunoglobulin may be advised to prevent or ameliorate congenital heart block.

Somewhere between 5,000 and 10,000 people in the United States have *childhood lupus*. Of these, 20% to 40% are male. Nearly 70% have organ-threatening disease, as opposed to 40% to 50% of adults. Special considerations are taken into account to minimize the use of drugs that interfere with growth and development, interact with an incomplete immune system, or influence potential fertility issues. Despite the severity of childhood lupus, mortality rates are surprisingly low and only slightly worse than with adult lupus.[2,6]

Adolescents with lupus have a high treatment nonadherence rate, especially with corticosteroids and other agents that alter mood, behavior, or appearance. Noncompliance with sun avoidance is also a problem. Fragile social relationships should not take second place to patients' being honest with their physician and family.

Lupus in the elderly is usually a milder, bland process that is more focused on musculoskeletal activity, constitutional symptoms, and Sjögren's-related signs. The symptoms are often difficult to differentiate from primary Sjögren's syndrome, rheumatoid arthritis (RA), or polymyalgia rheumatica. Only 2% of cases of lupus develop in patients over the age of 70. Organ-threatening disease is rare, and patients are frequently responsive to low doses of corticosteroids. Mortality studies suggest a poorer prognosis for lupus in older patients; in this author's opinion, it relates to non-lupus-associated comorbidities.

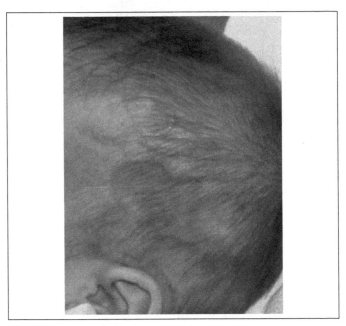

Figure 8.1 Neonatal lupus. ©1972–2004 American College of Rheumatology Clinical Slide Collection. Used with permission.

Overlapping Syndromes

Defined in Chapter 2, mixed connective tissue disease and overlap syndromes occur when a patient has another defined rheumatic process in addition to systemic lupus erythematosus. Once thought to be a benign process, MCTD has a 20-year mortality rate of over 50%. Patients should be screened for pulmonary hypertension, nutritional problems related to dysmotility or malabsorption, myositis, and malignant hypertension. Elevated titers of anti-RNP must be present by definition. One case of MCTD is reported for every 20 persons with SLE. Overlap syndrome patients lack anti-RNP and are managed in the same manner as patients with lupus and other rheumatic disease.

Undifferentiated Connective Tissue Disease

It has been estimated that lupus is the "tip of the iceberg" and that for every patient with SLE, seven patients have an undifferentiated connective tissue disease. Many report a spontaneous disappearance of the process, or a palindromic course where the symptoms wax and wane or signs disappear for months or years at a time. Nonsteroidal anti-inflammatory drugs, antimalarial therapies, and intermittent low-dose corticosteroids are usually effective. Of the one-third with UCTD who evolve an American College of Rheumatology–defined autoimmune processes, 70% develop RA and only 20% develop SLE.

Drug-Exacerbated and -Induced Lupus

Some patients with established lupus experience exacerbations of the disease when given certain agents. These agents include sulfa-containing drugs, nonsteroidal drugs, and tetracyclines, among others. It is thought that this occurs via a sun-sensitizing mechanism (see Table 8.1).[3]

Many drugs can induce a positive antinuclear antibody in some patients; only a small percentage of these patients ever develop a clinically evident lupus-like reaction. For only six agents is the development of SLE reported in at least 1 in 1000 users. They account for 90% of cases of drug-exacerbated and -induced

Table 8.1 Drug-exacerbated and -induced lupus: A partial list of causal agents

1. Drugs proven to induce clinical lupus in at least 1 of 1000 cases
   - Hydralazine
   - Procainamide
   - Methyldopa
   - D-penicillamine
   - Tumor necrosis factor (TNF) blockers
   - Minocycline
2. Drugs proven to induce clinical lupus in at least 1 of 10,000 cases
   - Isoniazid
   - Sulfasalazine
   - Carbamazepine
   - Phenothiazines
   - Quinidine
   - Griseofulvin
3. Drugs that infrequently exacerbate but do not cause lupus
   - Antibiotics (e.g., arylamine sulfas, tetracyclines)
   - Nonsteroidal anti-inflammatory drugs (e.g., ibuprofen, piroxicam)
   - Oral contraceptives and other hormones
4. Mechanisms of drug-induced lupus
   - Drug promotes autoreactive T cells (e.g., phenytoin)
   - Drug is sun-sensitizing (e.g., phenothiazines)
   - Drug alters DNA and renders it immunogenic (e.g., procainamide)
   - Metabolic breakdown products in slow acetylators are immunogenic (e.g., hydralazine)
   - Drugs promote altered DNA repair via hypomethylation
5. Drugs shown to induce subacute cutaneous lupus rashes
   - Thiazide diuretics
   - Cimetidine
   - Calcium channel blockers
   - Angiotensin-converting enzyme inhibitors

lupus and include hydralazine, procainamide, minocycline, tumor necrosis factor (TNF) inhibitors, methyldopa, and D-penicillamine. Organ-threatening disease is almost unheard of, and musculoskeletal, serositis, and constitutional presentations predominate. Resolution of the process occurs in over 90% within three months of discontinuation of the drug. Some of the patients given anti-TNF agents may have had lupus to begin with, because early lupus and RA are difficult to differentiate. Nonsteroidal drugs, salicylates, and low doses of corticosteroids may be needed in some patients and are very effective.

Antiphospholipid Syndrome

Defined in Chapter 2, 11% of persons with SLE have a hypercoagulable state. An equal number of patients without SLE develop the same process. A variety of factors allow lupus patients to be at an increased risk for developing thromboembolic disease, such as a protein cofactor to anti-β_2 glycoprotein, endothelial exposure, and aberrations in the prostacyclin pathway.[5] Over 90% of APS cases can be diagnosed by performing a specialized partial thromboplastin time, anti-β_2 glycoprotein, anticardiolipin antibody, and circulating anticoagulant. A list of proteins and antibodies found more commonly in SLE that are associated with thromboembolic events is given in Table 8.2. Higher titers of IgG isotype phospholipid antibodies increase thromboembolic risks. The overwhelming majority of patients with an antiphospholipid antibody never experience an event. However, some of these patients have recurrent miscarriages and are only at risk during pregnancy.

Patients deemed to be at high risk for a thromboembolic event but who have never had one may benefit from daily low-dose aspirin. Antiphospholipid syndrome (APS) patients should be on lifelong anticoagulation, usually in the form of warfarin. Warfarin resistance warrants low-molecular-weight heparin; patients with arterial events sometimes benefit from the addition of low-dose aspirin, clopidogrel, or dipyramidole.

One percent of APS patients sustain recurrent events despite adequate therapy. These patients have *catastrophic antiphospholipid syndrome* (CAPS). This serious complication has a 50% mortality rate within two years and mandates anti-inflammatory interventions as well (e.g., immunosuppressives, apheresis).

Pregnancy

Lupus patients are normally fertile. However, only 67% of pregnancies in SLE patients are successful, compared to 85% in the general population.[4] There are several contraindications to pregnancy wherein the life of the mother is jeopardized: myocarditis, renal failure, malignant hypertension, pulmonary hypertension, or recurrent thromboembolic events. Certain medications commonly used in SLE are also contraindicated. These include methotrexate, cyclophosphamide, mycophenolate mofetil, cyclosporine, angiotensin-converting enzyme inhibitors, warfarin, and rituximab. Antimalarial therapies are safe and decrease

Table 8.2 Clinical associations of anticardiolipin antibody

Immunology/rheumatology
- Antiphospholipid antibody syndrome
- Systemic lupus erythematosus
- Lupus anticoagulant
- Chronic biological false positive test for syphilis
- Rheumatoid arthritis
- Sjögren's syndrome
- Ulcerative colitis
- Behçet's syndrome
- Drug-induced lupus erythematosus
- Other autoimmune disorders

Obstetrics
- Recurrent fetal loss

Hematology
- Arterial and venous thrombosis
  Thrombocytopenia
  Coombs' positive hemolytic anemia
  Evan's syndrome

Neurology
- Cerebral thrombosis
- Transient ischemic attack
- Chorea
- Transverse myelopathy
- Epilepsy
- Migraine

Cardiology
- Libman Sacks endocarditis
- Coronary thrombosis
- Labile hypertension

Pulmonary
- Pulmonary emboli
- Pulmonary hypertension

Dermatology
- Livedo reticularis
- Digital gangrene
- Chronic leg ulcers

Miscellaneous
- Drugs
  - Chlorpromazine
  - Pronestyl
  - Others
- Infections
  - AIDS
  - Mononucleosis
  - Others
- Malignancies

pregnancy-related disease exacerbations. Corticosteroids and occasional non-steroidal anti-inflammatory drugs are permitted. Apheresis and intravenous immunoglobulin can be safely used if indicated.

Low-risk mothers are those with chronic cutaneous (discoid) lupus, drug-induced lupus, and non-organ-threatening disease with slight to no activity. Most pregnancy flares occur during the first trimester; afterward, the fetus, the placenta, and the mother's stressed adrenal gland make extra corticosteroids. Blood pressure, urinary protein, blood sugars, and weight should be carefully monitored. A drop in C3 complement is associated with increased disease activity and a poorer pregnancy outcome. The prevalence of preeclampsia is increased in SLE. APS patients usually benefit from low-molecular-weight heparin and low-dose aspirin. Low-dose aspirin should be discontinued at week 28 to allow the patent ductus arteriosus to close. After delivery, postpartum flares occur in as many as 30% of patients between weeks 2 and 8. Short or increased doses of corticosteroids usually are efficacious. Breastfeeding is usually allowed in those taking all permissible medications.

References

1. Izmirly PM, Rivera TL, Buyon JP. Neonatal lupus syndromes. *Rheum Dis Clin N Am.* 2007;33:267–285.

2. Arkachaisri T, Lehman TL. Systemic lupus erythematosus and related disorders of childhood. *Curr Opin Rheumatol.* 1999;11:384–392.

3. Vasoo S. Drug-induced lupus erythematosus: an update. *Lupus.* 2006;15:757–761.

4. Clowse ME. Lupus activity in pregnancy. *Rheum Dis Clin N Am.* 2007;33:237–252.

5. Bertolaccini ML, Khamashta MA, Hughes GR. Diagnosis of antiphospholipid syndrome. *Nat Clin Prac Rheumatol.* 2005;1:40–46.

6. Lehman TJA. SLE in childhood and adolescence. In: DJ Wallace and BH Hahn. *Dubois' Lupus Erythematosus and Related Disorders*, 8th ed. Philadelphia, PA: Elsevier; 2013:495–505.

Chapter 9

Methods of Clinical Ascertainment

The American College of Rheumatology criteria and SLICC criteria for the classification of SLE apply to epidemiological surveys and inclusion in clinical trials. Patients can have lupus without fulfilling the criteria. Physicians use a variety of parameters to make clinical decisions regarding lupus patients.[4–6] These include the following:

- Symptoms (e.g., stiffness, aching, fatigue)
- Signs (e.g., rashes, synovitis)
- Laboratory abnormalities (e.g., anemia, elevated sedimentation rate)
- Serological abnormalities (e.g., elevated anti-DNA)
- Electrical abnormalities (e.g., EKG [ECG], EEG, EMG)
- Imaging abnormalities (e.g., chest radiograph, 2-D echocardiography, computed tomography scanning, or magnetic resonance imaging)

In 2010, the U.S. Food and Drug Administration issued a Guidance Document, which provided a guide to clinical investigators for clinical trials.[1] Among its recommendations the document relates that the following factors are acceptable means for demonstrating the efficacy and safety of a specific intervention:

- The drug is safe.
- Quality of life is improved (e.g., Lupus PRO).
- A validated clinical index demonstrates less disease activity (e.g., the BILAG and either the SLEDAI or the SLAM)[2,3] (Fig. 9.1, Table 9.1). The Systemic Lupus Erythematosus Disease Activity Index (SLEDAI) takes less than a minute to calculate; the majority of its values relate to the central nervous and renal systems. It fails to include many manifestations of the disease and deemphasizes laboratory abnormalities. The British Isles Lupus Assessment Group (BILAG) is extremely complex and thorough but is not subject to consistently reliable statistical analysis, while the Systemic Lupus Activity Measure (SLAM) includes subjective components. Hence, most clinical trial designs utilize at least two of these metrics.
- A response measure demonstrates improvement (e.g., the SLE Responder Index) (Fig. 9.2).[6]
- There is less advancement of scarring or damage (e.g., SLICC/ACR Damage Index).[4]
- Trials should be of one year duration in patients stratified by severity, with flares, responses, and steroid sparing carefully defined.
- There are organ-specific measures (e.g., CLASI for cutaneous disease,[5] renal indices).
- No surrogate markers or biomarkers are yet acceptable in ascertaining and following disease activity, but promising prospects (e.g., the interferon signature) could be acceptable metrics to shorten the length of clinical trials.

CHAPTER 9 **Methods of Clinical Ascertainment**
68

BILAG2004 INDEX   Centre: Date: Initials/Hosp No:

Only record items **due to SLE Disease Activity** & assessment refers to manifestations occurring in the **last 4 weeks** (compared with the previous 4 weeks).   ♦♦ **TO BE USED WITH THE GLOSSARY** ♦♦

Scoring   ND   Not Done
          1   Improving
          2   Same
          3   Worse
          4   New
          Yes/No OR Value (where indicated)
          ❑ indicate if **not due to SLE activity**
          (default is 0 = not present)

CONSTITUTIONAL
1. Pyrexia - documented > 37.5°C ( )
2. Weight loss - unintentional > 5% ( )
3. Lymphadenopathy/splenomegaly ( )
4. Anorexia ( )

MUCOCUTANEOUS
5. Skin eruption - severe ( )
6. Skin eruption - mild ( )
7. Angio-oedema - severe ( )
8. Angio-oedema - mild ( )
9. Mucosal ulceration - severe ( )
10. Mucosal ulceration - mild ( )
11. Panniculitis/Bullous lupus - severe ( )
12. Panniculitis/Bullous lupus - mild ( )
13. Major cutaneous vasculitis/thrombosis ( )
14. Digital infarcts or nodular vasculitis ( )
15. Alopecia - severe ( )
16. Alopecia - mild ( )
17. Peri-ungual erythema/chilblains ( )
18. Splinter haemorrhages ( )

NEUROPSYCHIATRIC
19. Aseptic meningitis ( )
20. Cerebral vasculitis ( )
21. Demyelinating syndrome ( )
22. Myelopathy ( )
23. Acute confusional state ( )
24. Psychosis ( )
25. Acute inflammatory demyelinating polyradiculoneuropathy ( )
26. Mononeuropathy (single/multiplex) ( )
27. Cranial neuropathy ( )
28. Plexopathy ( )
29. Polyneuropathy ( )
30. Seizure disorder ( )
31. Status epilepticus ( )
32. Cerebrovascular disease (not due to vasculitis) ( )
33. Cognitive dysfunction ( )
34. Movement disorder ( )
35. Autonomic disorder ( )
36. Cerebellar ataxia (isolated) ( )
37. Lupus headache - severe unremitting ( )
38. Headache from IC hypertension ( )

MUSCULOSKELETAL
39. Myositis - severe ( )
40. Myositis - mild ( )
41. Arthritis (severe) ( )
42. Arthritis (moderate)/Tendonitis/Tenosynovitis ( )
43. Arthritis (mild)/Arthralgia/Myalgia ( )

Weight (kg):   Serum urea (mmol/l):
African ancestry: Yes/No   Serum albumin (g/l):

CARDIORESPIRATORY
44. Myocarditis - mild ( )
45. Myocarditis/Endocarditis + Cardiac failure ( )
46. Arrhythmia ( )
47. New valvular dysfunction ( )
48. Pleurisy/Pericarditis ( )
49. Cardiac tamponade ( )
50. Pleural effusion with dyspnoea ( )
51. Pulmonary haemorrhage/vasculitis ( )
52. Interstitial alveolitis/pneumonitis ( )
53. Shrinking lung syndrome ( )
54. Aortitis ( )
55. Coronary vasculitis ( )

GASTROINTESTINAL
56. Lupus peritonitis ( )
57. Abdominal serositis or ascites ( )
58. Lupus enteritis/colitis ( )
59. Malabsorption ( )
60. Protein losing enteropathy ( )
61. Intestinal pseudo-obstruction ( )
62. Lupus hepatitis ( )
63. Acute lupus cholecystitis ( )
64. Acute lupus pancreatitis ( )

OPHTHALMIC
65. Orbital inflammation/myositis/proptosis ( )
66. Keratitis - severe ( )
67. Keratitis - mild ( )
68. Anterior uveitis ( )
69. Posterior uveitis/retinal vasculitis - severe ( )
70. Posterior uveitis/retinal vasculitis - mild ( )
71. Episcleritis ( )
72. Scleritis - severe ( )
73. Scleritis - mild ( )
74. Retinal/choroidal vaso-occlusive disease ( )
75. Isolated cotton-wool spots (cytoid bodies) ( )
76. Optic neuritis ( )
77. Anterior ischaemic optic neuropathy ( )

RENAL
78. Systolic blood pressure (mm Hg)   value ( ) ❑
79. Diastolic blood pressure (mm Hg)   value ( ) ❑
80. Accelerated hypertension   Yes/No ( )
81. Urine dipstick protein (=1, ==2, ===3) ( ) ❑
82. Urine albumin-creatinine ratio   mg/mmol ( ) ❑
83. Urine protein-creatinine ratio   mg/mmol ( ) ❑
84. 24 hour urine protein (g)   value ( ) ❑
85. Nephrotic syndrome   Yes/No ( )
86. Creatinine (plasma/serum)   μmol/l ( ) ❑
87. GFR (calculated)   ml/min/1.73 m² ( ) ❑
88. Active urinary sediment   Yes/No ( )
89. Active nephritis   Yes/No ( )

HAEMATOLOGICAL
90. Haemoglobin (g/dl)   value ( ) ❑
91. Total white cell count (x 10⁹/l)   value ( ) ❑
92. Neutrophils (x 10⁹/l)   value ( ) ❑
93. Lymphocytes (x 10⁹/l)   value ( ) ❑
94. Platelets (x 10⁹/l)   value ( ) ❑
95. TTP ( )
96. Evidence of active haemolysis   Yes/No ( )
97. Coombs' test positive (isolated)   Yes/No ( )

Investigator Signature: _____   Date: _____

Figure 9.1 The 2004 British Isles Lupus Assessment Group (BILAG) checksheet form. This version of the form is the one currently used in most ongoing clinical trials.

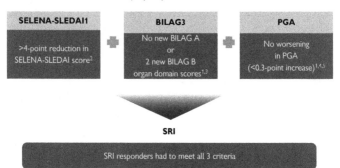

Primary Endpoint: SLE Responder Index
(SRI) Response Rate at Week 52

SELENA-SLEDAI1 — >4-point reduction in SELENA-SLEDAI score[2]

BILAG3 — No new BILAG A or 2 new BILAG B organ domain scores[1,3]

PGA — No worsening in PGA (<0.3-point increase)[1,4,5]

SRI

SRI responders had to meet all 3 criteria

SELENA-SLEDAI=Safety of Estrogens in Lupus Erythematosus: National Assessment Version of the Systemic Lupus Erythematosus Disease Activity Index; BILAG=British Isles Lupus Assessment Group; PGA=Physician's Global Assessment

Figure 9.2 The SLE Responder Index.[6]

Table 9.1 SELENA-SLEDAI Index

Weight	Descriptor	Definition
8	Seizure	Recent onset (last 10 days). Exclude metabolic, infectious drug cause, or seizure due to past irreversible CNS damage.
8	Psychosis	Altered ability to function in normal activity due to severe disturbance in the perception of reality. Include hallucinations, incoherence, marked loose associations, impoverished thought content, marked illogical thinking, bizarre, disorganized, or catatonic behavior. Exclude uremia and drug causes.
8	Organic Brain Syndrome	Altered mental function with impaired orientation, memory, or other intellectual function, with rapid onset and fluctuating clinical features. Include clouding of consciousness with reduced capacity to focus and inability to sustain attention to environment, plus at least 2 of the following: perceptual disturbance, incoherent speech, insomnia or daytime drowsiness, or increased or decreased psychomotor activity. Exclude metabolic, infectious, or drug causes.
8	Visual Disturbance	Retinal and eye changes of SLE. Include cytoid bodies, retinal hemorrhages, serious exudate of hemorrhage in the choroid, optic neuritis, seleritis, or episcleritis. Exclude hypertension, infection, or drug causes.
8	Cranial Nerve Disorder	New onset sensory or motor neuropathy involving cranial nerves. Include vertigo due to lupus.
8	Lupus Headache	Severe persistent headache: may be migrainous, but must be non-responsive to narcotic analgesia.
8	Cerebrovascular Accident (CVA)	New onset of CVA(s). Exclude arteriosclerosis or hypertensive causes.
8	Vasculitis	Ulceration, gangrene, tender finger nodules, periungual infarction, splinter hemorrhages, or biopsy or angiogram proof of vasculitis.
4	Arthritis	More than 2 joints with pain & signs of inflammation (i.e., tenderness, swelling or effusion).
4	Myositis	Proximal muscle aching/weakness associated with elevated creatine phosphokinase/aldolase or electromyogram changes or a biopsy showing myositis.
4	Urinary Casts	Heme-granular or red blood cell casts.
4	Hematuria	>5 red blood cells/high power field. Exclude stone, infection, or other causes.
4	Proteinuria	New onset or recent increase of more than 0.5 g/24 hours.
4	Pyuria	>5 white blood cells/high power field. Exclude infection.
2	Rash	New or ongoing inflammatory lupus rash.

(continued)

Table 9.1 (Continued)

Weight	Descriptor	Definition
2	Alopecia	New or ongoing abnormal, patchy or diffuse loss of hair due to active lupus.
2	Mucosal Ulcers	New or ongoing oral or nasal ulcerations due to active lupus.
2	Pleurisy	Classic and severe pleuritic chest pain or pleural rub or effusion or new pleural thickening due to lupus.
2	Pericarditis	Classic and severe pericardial pain or rub or effusion, or electrocardiogram confirmation.
2	Low Complement	Decrease in CH50, C3, or C4 below the lower limit of normal for testing laboratory.
2	Increased DNA Binding	>25% binding by Farr assay or above normal range for testing laboratory.
1	Fever	>38°C. Exclude infectious cause.
1	Thrombocytopenia	<100,000 platelets/mm3
1	Leukopenia	<3,000 white blood cells/mm3. Exclude drug causes.
	TOTAL SCORE	**(Sum of weights next to descriptors marked present)**

Score if descriptor is present at time of visit or in the preceding 10 days.
SLEDAI—Systemic Lupus Erythematosus Disease Activity Index
SELENA—Selective use of Estrogens in Lupus Erythematosus National Assessment

Lupologists are in the process of reconfiguring how they follow their patients and what parameters are used in the clinic on the basis of information derived from clinical trials.

References

1. U.S. Food and Drug Administration. *Guidance for Industry on Systemic Lupus Erythematosus: Developing Medical Products for Treatment.* Available at http://www.fda.gov/Drugs/GuidanceComplianceRegulatoryInformation/Guidances/UCM07263.pdf. Accessed March 11, 2013.

2. Gladman DD, Ibañez D, Urowitz MB. Systemic lupus erythematosus disease activity index 2000. *J Rheumatol.* 2002;29:288–291.

3. Yee CS, Farewell V, Isenberg DA, et al. British Isles Lupus Assessment Group 2004 index is valid for assessment of disease activity in systemic lupus erythematosus. *Arthritis Rheum.* 2007;56:4113–4119.

4. Gladman DD, Goldsmith CH, Urowitz MB, et al. The Systemic Lupus International Collaborating Clinics/American College of Rheumatology (SLICC/ACR) Damage Index for Systemic Lupus Erythematosus International Comparison. *J Rheumatol.* 2000;27:373–376.

5. Klein R, Moghadam-Kia S, LoMonico J, et al. Development of the CLASI as a tool to measure disease activity and responsiveness to therapy in cutaneous lupus erythematosus. *Arch Dermatol.* 2011 Feb;147(2):203–208.

6. Furie RA, Petri MA, Wallace DJ, et al. Novel evidence-based systemic lupus erythematosus responder index. *Arthritis Rheum.* 2009 Sep 15;61(9):1143–1151.

Chapter 10

General Treatment Concepts

Lupus patients can help themselves improve their disease by initiating life-style changes that, in controlled studies, diminish morbidity and mortality (Table 10.1).[1]

Physical Measures and Exercise

Sun avoidance is advised. Outdoor activities should be undertaken in the early morning, late afternoon, or early evening. Individuals living at sea level get less ultraviolet exposure than those at higher altitudes. Sun-protective clothing is available for purchase from several Web sites. Table 10.2 contains a list of sunscreens that block ultraviolet A and B light. Painful joints respond to moist heat. Changes in barometric pressure may increase stiffness or aching. Fatigue is managed with pacing, alternating periods of activity with rest. Restful sleep is important. Physical and occupational therapists can teach patients how to maximize their body mechanics, perform an evaluation of activities of daily living, recommend ergonomic saving measures, and promote the use of assistive devices. Exercise diminishes inflammation and steroid-induced muscular atrophy and demineralization. Inflamed joints should not be isotonically exercised, but range-of-motion activities decrease risks for contractures and deformity. Pilates-based stretching and isometric-based strengthening are recommended, along with walking and low-impact aerobics. If fibromyalgia is present, weight-lifting, rowing, tennis, bowling, and golf should be restricted, as they tend to increase upper back and neck discomfort.[3]

Diet

The "lupus diet" is a well-balanced diet. Alfalfa sprouts may aggravate lupus; fish and fish oil supplements have anti-inflammatory properties. Individuals on corticosteroids should adopt a diabetic and antihypertensive diet with salt, cholesterol, and carbohydrate restriction. Protein restriction is recommended with advanced renal disease.

Managing Fatigue and Smoking

Fatigue is reported in over 90% of persons with systemic lupus erythematosus and can result from inflammation, depression, medications, comorbidities (e.g., anemia, hypothyroidism), or fibromyalgia, among other factors.[2] The cause or causes of fatigue need to be delineated. Treatment measures include pacing,

Table 10.1 Non-lupus medication measures shown to have a favorable evidence based impact upon lupus[5]

1. Educating patients about the disease
2. A well-balanced diet, especially one that restricts carbohydrate and fat intake in patients taking corticosteroids
3. Aerobic exercise
4. Being up to date with immunizations
5. Smoking cessation
6. Being compliant with appointments and adherent with medication regimens
7. Stress-reduction measures
8. Establishing a coordinated primary care/lupus specialist interface to ensure health maintenance standards
9. Screening for accelerated atherogenesis
10. Bone density measurements when appropriate
11. Sun protection measures

an exercise program, and optimal sleep hygiene for managing the source of fatigue.[3] Smoking worsens Raynaud's phenomenon and diminishes aerobic capacity, which further aggravates fatigue and interferes with the efficacy of antimalarial therapies.[4]

Psychosocial Support

Emotional stress flares autoimmune disease in animal models, and many patients experience more symptoms while experiencing psychosocial stressors. Coping is often difficult because of fears, anxiety, anger, pain, or depression. Additionally, patients may not look sick, and physician–patient relationships can be suboptimal. Patients are encouraged to develop concrete goals and positive attitudes, optimize their family environment, and seek counseling where appropriate. Cognitive-behavioral therapy, biofeedback, and stress-reduction strategies have been shown to improve coping mechanisms in evidence-based studies.

Table 10.2 Sun protection and safe sun habits

1. Schedule outdoor activities before 10 AM and after 4 PM
2. Up to 80% of ultraviolet (UV) light penetrates cloud cover and can be reflected from water, concrete, sand, snow, tile, and reflective glass in buildings. Extra care is important at higher altitudes.
3. Clothing is an excellent form of sun protection, especially loose-fitting, lightweight dark clothing, sunglasses, and broad-brimmed hats.
4. Protective clothing for UV-B light with a sun protective factor of 30 or higher. Sunblocks should be applied 15–20 minutes before sun exposure and can be liberally applied. UV-A protection is also desirable. Do not apply to broken skin or rashes.
5. UV-B sunblocks with avobenzone and zinc oxide also block UV-A1, and titanium dioxide are the best for very sensitive skin.
6. Sunblocks are available as creams, lotions, gels, sprays, sticks, in waterproof and heat-resistant forms as well as in lip and eyelid formulations.

Adjunctive Measures: Osteoporosis, Allergies, Vaccinations, and Antibiotics

Inflammation from SLE demineralizes bones, as do corticosteroids and methotrexate, among other agents. Lupus patients should undergo bone density screening at regular intervals. Bisphosphonates are the agent of choice for those at risk; raloxifene is contraindicated in some due to its thrombotic potential. Individuals with SLE have the same to a slightly increased risk for allergies compared with the general population. A minority may flare with immunotherapy, and this intervention should only be used if other measures fail and it is closely followed. Live vaccinations are usually contraindicated in lupus patients unless they are in a total remission off medication. Patients who are immunosuppressed have a normal to decreased response to killed vaccines. Post-immunization disease flares are infrequent, but they do occur. Sulfa-based antibiotics with an arylamine component (e.g., sulfamethoxasole) are sun-sensitizing and should be avoided. Minocyclines may flare lupus as well, but doxycyclines are safe. Dental antibiotic prophylaxis is advisable in immunosuppressed patients or those with antiphospholipid syndrome.

References

1. Wallace DJ. Principles of therapy and local measures. In: DJ Wallace, BH Hahn, eds. *Dubois' Lupus Erythematosus.* 7th ed. Philadelphia, PA: Lippincott Williams & Wilkins; 2007:1132–1134.

2. Ad Hoc Committee on Systemic Lupus Erythematosus Response Criteria for Fatigue. Measurement of fatigue in systemic lupus erythematosus: a systemic review, *Arthritis Care Res.* 2003;57:1348–1357.

3. Robb-Nicholson LC, Daltroy L, Eaton H, et al. Effects of aerobic conditioning in lupus fatigue: a pilot study. *Br J Rheumatol.* 1989; 28:500–505.

4. Ghaussy NO, Sibbitt W Jr, Bankhurst AD, Qualls CR. Cigarette smoking and disease activity in systemic lupus erythematosus. *J Rheumatol.* 2003;30:1215–1221.

5. Wallace DJ. Improving the prognosis of SLE without prescribing lupus drugs and the primary care paradox. *Lupus.* 2008;17:91–92.

Chapter 11

Medications Used to Manage Lupus Erythematosus

The pharmacological treatment of lupus revolves around four considerations[1]:

1. Is there organ-threatening disease (cardiopulmonary, hepatic, renal, hematological, central nervous system) that requires corticosteroids and immunosuppressive therapy?
2. Is there non-organ-threatening disease (constitutional, musculoskeletal, cutaneous, serositis) warranting disease-modifying therapy?
3. Should organ-specific measures (e.g., treatment of a rash) be implemented?
4. Which adjunctive treatments (e.g., bisphosphonates, angiotensin-converting enzyme inhibitors) are appropriate for the patient?

The principles of drug therapy for lupus state that organ-threatening disease should be managed aggressively with moderate to high doses of corticosteroids, often followed by the institution of steroid-sparing measures in the form of immunosuppressives. Antimalarials are usually introduced as well. Non-organ-threatening disease is managed with nonsteroidal anti-inflammatory drugs (NSAIDs), antimalarials, and low doses of steroids if necessary.

Nonsteroidal Anti-inflammatory Agents and Salicylates

The safest NSAID from a cardioprotective standpoint is naproxen, with or without a proton-pump inhibitor. All other NSAIDs are acceptable in lupus, but with certain caveats: celecoxib is gentler on the stomach and safer in patients on warfarin but has a sulfa component, ibuprofen is associated with infrequent aseptic meningitis, and others (e.g., piroxicam) are sun-sensitizing. These agents are useful for headaches, fevers, serositis, arthralgia, arthritis, myalgias, and generalized pain. They do not have disease-modifying properties. NSAIDs are as efficacious as, and easier to use than, salicylates.

Antimalarials

Chloroquine, hydroxychloroquine, and quinacrine (available from compounding pharmacists) prevent the activation of Toll receptors 7 and 9 and raise cellular pH, which turns off receptor activation sites. They have been used in lupus for over 50 years and are approved by the Food and Drug Administration for this indication. Hydroxychloroquine is the agent of choice. It can diminish the risk of non-organ dissemination in mild disease, decrease the rate of disease flares, and prevent damage accrual; it is approved for use in rheumatoid arthritis (RA) and thus treats synovitis, and it has ameliorative effects on all aspects of organ-threatening disease (especially cutaneous) (Fig. 11.1). Given in doses of 5 to 7 mg/kg, hydroxychloroquine (Plaquenil) begins working in 6 to 12 weeks but does not attain its maximal effects for up to 6 months.[2] Recent work suggests that antimalarials also lower cholesterol levels, inhibit platelet aggregation, and improve sicca symptoms associated with Sjögren's syndrome. Retrospecive studies have associated hydroxychloroquine with less damage accrual, prolonged survival, better renal and skin outcomes, delay in disease onset, less vascular damage, fewer infections and thromboembolic events, and lower blood pressure in lupus patients.[7]

Ten percent report flu-like symptoms, gastrointestinal distress, or a headache with hydroxychloroquine; this rate is lower when generic preparations are not prescribed. Of those who take the drug for 10 years, 3% develop a reversible maculopathy. Annual ophthalmological examinations are advised after an initial evaluation and at five years in individuals with specific risk factors.[8]

Chloroquine is very effective for severe cutaneous disease in doses of 500 mg/day for 30 days followed by 250 mg/day for 3 months. Commonly used in developing countries due to its minimal cost, it is more retinotoxic than other treatments (10% develop changes in 10 years, and these may not always be reversible). Most patients who respond to chloroquine are transitioned to hydroxychloroquine for maintenance.

Quinacrine is synergistic with the chloroquines, is effective for cutaneous lupus, and diminishes fatigue. It is not toxic to the eyes. It produces a yellowish

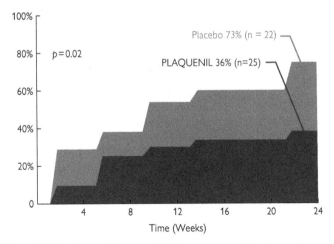

Figure 11.1 The Canadian Cooperative Trial documentation of the efficacy of hydroxychloroquine (Plaquenil) in preventing lupus flares. *Source: N Engl J Med.* 1991;324:150-154.

stain, and 30% of patients taking it develop mild diarrhea. Quinacrine is dosed at 50 to 100 mg/day, and a complete blood count and basic metabolic panel should be obtained quarterly (Table 11.1).

Corticosteroids

The use of corticosteroids is a critical intervention in managing systemic lupus. Patients with organ-threatening disease are usually prescribed 1 mg/kg/day prednisone equivalent for 4 to 6 weeks followed by tapering by 10% per week. Flares of synovitis, rashes, fevers, or serositis are managed with lower doses for days to weeks. Patients with non-organ-threatening disease rarely require maintenance doses of greater than 15 mg/day. The long-term use of corticosteroids is associated with premature atherogenesis, hyperlipidemia, hyperglycemia, cataracts, glaucoma, emotional lability, bone demineralization, ecchymosis, peptic ulcer disease, and avascular necrosis (Table 11.2).

Immunosuppressive Regimens

If patients with organ-threatening lupus demonstrate active disease on 10 mg of prednisone equivalent or less, an immunosuppressant is usually introduced. The same concept applies to patients on lower doses if there are additional risk factors present such as diabetes or difficulty tolerating corticosteroid therapy. The principal immunosuppressants used in SLE are discussed next.

Methotrexate is an antimetabolite that inhibits dehydrofolate reductase and promotes adenosine release. It is effective for synovitis and some constitutional and cutaneous manifestations of SLE but is not helpful for organ involvement. The dosing is similar to that used in RA (10 to 20 mg weekly with 1 mg/day of folic acid).

Table 11.1 Antimalarials for lupus erythematosus
1. Principal relevant effects
a. Inhibits phospholipase A2 and phospholipase C
b. Stabilization of lysosomal membranes
c. Decreased production of estrogen
d. Quinidine-like cardiac effects
e. Antagonism of Toll-like receptors (TLR-7 and 9)
f. Photoprotection
2. Evidence-based clinical effects of hydroxychloroquine
a. Sustained beneficial effect on overall survival, disease-free survival, and damage accrual
b. Delayed onset of SLE and flare rate reduction
c. Protection against thromboembolic events
d. Protective effect against renal damage
e. Decreases in infection rate
f. Lowering of blood sugar and improvement in lipid profiles

Wallace DJ, Gudsoorkar VS, Weisman MH et al. New insights into mechanisms of therapeutic effects of antimalarial agents in SLE. *Nature Rev Rheumatol.* 2012;8:522–533.

Table 11.2 Corticosteroids for SLE

1. Available preparations:
   a. Pulse intravenous methylprednisolone—given for life- or organ-threatening complications and severe flares in doses of 1G daily for 1–5 days. Oral methylprednisolone—preferred in children due to its advantages in an immature liver; does well in adults
   b. Prednisone—the gold standard
   c. Betamethasone—available intramuscular, intraarticular and topically; crosses the placenta
   d. Triamcinolone—available intramuscular and topically
   e. Hydrocortisone—available topically, orally (short half-life; used for rapid induction but is salt-retaining; used intravenously in emergency crises as it is effective within 20 minutes)
   f. Dexamethasone—available as topical, intraarticular, intramuscular, or oral preparations. May be useful for central nervous system disease
2. Usual regimens for systemic disease:
   a. Pulse steroids (see above)
   b. High-dose prednisone equivalent (30–100 mg daily), used for at least a month for life- or organ-threatening complications (e.g., nephritis, pneumonitis, central nervous system vasculitis, autoimmune hemolytic anemia, retinitis)
   c. Moderate dose prednisone equivalent (7.5–30 mg daily), used for myositis, pleurisy, thrombocytopenia, for example
   d. Low dose prednisone equivalent (<7.5 mg daily) is used for arthritis, mild constitutional symptoms, maintenance therapy, rashes, for example.
   e. Alternate day prednisone equivalent is used as chronic maintenance therapy where hypothalamic-pituitary-axis sparing is a goal (e.g., membranous nephritis)

Leflunomide is a pyrimidine antagonist. Dosing is 20 mg/day after a 3-day loading dose of 100 mg, and it is used for the same indications as methotrexate.

Azathioprine is an antimetabolite purine antagonist approved by the U.S. Food and Drug Administration, previously approved for RA, and is effective for synovitis. Controlled studies have also demonstrated efficacy for nephritis and hepatic involvement. Case series have demonstrated that it is useful in managing hematological, pulmonary, myositis, and cutaneous manifestations of the disease. Patients are usually started at 50 mg/day for the first week, 100 mg/day for the second week, and 150 mg/day maintenance. Lower doses can be used if there is gastrointestinal intolerance or in patients with stable disease after several years. Ten percent and 1% of patients are heterozygous or homozygous, respectively, for thiopurine S-methyltransferase enzyme activity and may have reactions to the drug. This can be prescreened for with an assay. The drug takes 3 to 4 months to become effective. Blood counts and liver function testing should be monitored every 1 to 3 months. After 3 years of therapy, there is an increased risk for lymphoma.

Mycophenolate mofetil inhibits inosine monophosphate dehydrogenase, which blocks B and T-cell proliferation. It is clearly beneficial for most forms of lupus nephritis. It is generally well tolerated, but up to 20% of patients are have difficulty taking it due to gastrointestinal complaints. Its administration for other manifestations of SLE has not been adequately studied or is not useful (e.g., with synovitis). Most patients are started at 500 mg/day and built up to a maintenance dose of 1500 to 3000 mg/day.

Cyclosporin is an immunosuppressant that inhibits interleukin-2. It is used for membranous nephritis and bone marrow hypoplasias or aplasia. Cyclosporin may be useful in certain refractory rashes seen in SLE. The usual dose is 3 mg/kg/day in divided doses.

Cyclophosphamide is a very powerful alkylating agent that is clearly effective for proliferative and membranous nephritis, central nervous system vasculitis, and serious pulmonary or hematological manifestations of the disease. Best given intravenously in doses of 750 mg/kg monthly for at least 6 months (NIH regimen or EUROLUPUS regimen of 500 mg every two weeks x 6 doses) followed by discontinuation or dosing every 2 to 3 months, this agent produces nausea and cytopenias.[3] The 80% risk of infertility in women receiving the drug over the age of 30 can be minimized by leuprolide injections (3.75 mg SC) 2 weeks prior to each dose (Fig. 11.2).

Nitrogen mustard was widely used in the mid 1900s for serious lupus but has been replaced by cyclophosphamide. *Chlorambucil* is ameliorative for renal disease but is leukemogenic and should not be used. *Tacrolimus* and *sirilimus* are transplant rejection drugs that have been safely given to lupus patients, and they are currently being studied for other aspects of the disease.

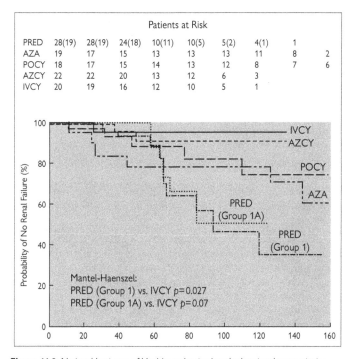

Figure 11.2 National Institutes of Health randomized study showing the superiority of cyclophosphamide for lupus nephritis over azathioprine or prednisone alone. *Source:* Balow JE, Austin HA 3rd, Tsokos GC, Antonovych TT, Steinberg AD, Klippel JH. NIH conference. Lupus nephritis. *Ann Intern Med.* 1987;106:79–94. ©1991 American College of Physicians. Reprinted with permission.

Other niche therapies are discussed earlier in this text under specific organ system manifestations.

Management of Organ- and Symptom-Specific Manifestations of Lupus

Constitutional

Lupus fever is acutely treated with NSAIDs, and corticosteroids if needed. Prednisone is the drug of choice and is usually given every 8 to 12 hours in doses of at least 0.25 kg/day. Hydrocortisone has a more rapid onset of action and can be used intravenously or orally every 6 hours in an emergency setting.

Cutaneous

Topical or Local Regimens

In addition to sunscreens, local measures include corticosteroids and immunosuppressants. Topical steroids include creams, ointments, and lotions and range from low to high potency. Over-the-counter topicals are nonfluorinated and contain hydrocortisone. Fluorinated corticosteroids are more powerful, but chronic use (especially on the face) can lead to cutaneous atrophy and telangiectasias. Facial use should be limited to no more than 2 weeks of treatment at a time. Creams are well tolerated but only 20% absorbed, as opposed to lotions (50%) and ointments (80%). Ointments are the most effective vehicle but are not tolerated as well and tend to be goopy and uncomfortable, especially with certain clothing (see Table 11.2). Where indicated, steroids may be injected intralesionally. On occasion, occlusive corticosteroid dressings are applied to refractory rashes. Pinecrolimus cream and tacrolimus ointments are approved in the United States for eczema, and these immunophylles are modestly effective for cutaneous lupus (see Table 11.3).

Acute Cutaneous Lupus

These lesions respond to systemic steroids, and the length and duration of therapy depend on how active extracutaneous manifestations of the disease are.

Chronic Cutaneous Lupus Erythematosus (Discoid Lupus)

In addition to topical and local regimens (see previous sections), antimalarials represent the gold standard for managing all except the mildest cases. Hydroxychloroquine is initiated in doses of 5 mg/kg/day and has a 6- to 12-week onset of action. More active lesions can be managed with up to 7 mg/kg/day of the drug for the first 3 months, or chloroquine can be substituted (500 mg/day). Upon improvement, these patients can usually be stabilized on 5 mg/kg/day hydroxychloroquine. Quinacrine can be added to the chloroquines and is synergistic (50 to 100 mg/day), or it can be used as monotherapy in individuals who cannot tolerate the chloroquines. Rarely used third-line agents include dapsone, retinoids, lamprene, and topical nitrogen mustard.

Table 11.3 Topical corticosteroids ranked by potency

Group	Generic name	Brand name
I. Superpotent	Clobetasol propionate cream, ointment, gel, or emollient, 0.05%	Temovate Diprolene
	Betamethasone dipropionate cream or ointment, 0.05%	Psorcon Ultravate
	Diflorasone diacetate ointment, 0.05%	
	Halobetasol propionate cream or ointment, 0.05%	
II. Potent	Amcinonide ointment, 0.1%	Cyclocort
	Betamethasone dipropionate cream, 0.05%	Diprolene
	Betamethasone dipropionate ointment, 0.05%	Diprolene Topicort
	Desoximetasone cream or ointment, 0.25%, and gel, 0.05%	Maxiflor Lidex Halog Elocon
	Diflorasone diacetate ointment, 0.05%	
	Fluocinonide cream, gel, or ointment, 0.05%	
	Halcinonide cream, 0.1%	
	Mometasone furoate ointment, 0.1%	
III. Midpotent	Amcinonide cream or lotion, 0.1%	Cyclocort
	Betamethasone dipropionate cream, 0.05%	Diprosone Valisone
	Betamethasone valerate ointment, 0.1%	Maxiflor Lidex-E
	Diflorasone diacetate cream, 0.05%	Cutivate Halog
	Fluocinonide cream, 0.05%	Aristocort A
	Fluticasone propionate ointment, 0.005%	
	Halcinonide ointment, 0.1%	
	Triamcinolone acetonide ointment, 0.1%	
IV. Midpotent	Fluocinolone acetonide ointment, 0.025%	Synalar Cordran
	Flurandrenolide ointment, 0.05%	Westcort Elocon
	Hydrocortisone valerate ointment, 0.2%	Kenalog
	Mometasone furoate cream, 0.1%	
	Triamcinolone acetonide cream, 0.1%	
V. Midpotent	Betamethasone dipropionate lotion, 0.05% Betamethasone valerate cream, 0.1%	Diprosone Valisone Synalar Cordran
	Fluocinolone acetonide cream, 0.025%	Cutivate Locoid
	Flurandrenolide cream, 0.05%	Westcort Kenalog
	Fluticasone propionate cream, 0.05%	
	Hydrocortisone butyrate cream, 0.05%	
	Hydrocortisone valerate cream, 0.2%	
	Triamcinolone acetonide lotion, 0.1%	
VI. Mild VII. Mild	Alclometasone dipropionate cream or ointment, 0.05%	Alcovate Valisone DesOwen
	Betamethasone valerate lotion, 0.05%	Locorten Synalar
	Desonide cream, 0.05%	Aristocort A
	Flumethasone pivalate cream, 0.03%	
	Fluocinolone acetonide cream or solution, 0.01% Triamcinolone acetonide cream, 0.1%	
	Topicals with hydrocortisone, dexamethasone, flumethasone, prednisolone, and methylprednisolone	

See copyright page of this book for permission to reprint Table 11.3.

Subacute Cutaneous Lupus

This lesion is not as responsive to the chloroquines as is discoid lupus. The addition of a retinoid (e.g., Soriatene, Accutane) for several weeks to months may be necessary.

Mucocutaneous Lesions

Oral ulcers are managed with buttermilk gargles, gargles of hydrogen peroxide diluted in water, or dental pastes containing corticosteroids. Nasal ulcerations are less frequent but need to be distinguished from Wegener's granulomatosis or the effects of cocaine use. Petroleum jelly (e.g., Vaseline) may be useful. Vaginal ulcerations are observed in 5% of females with SLE at some point in the course of their disease. Cyclosporin can ameliorate chronic aphthous stomatitis.

Alopecia

Reducing inflammation is the best treatment, and alopecia is often the last manifestation of the disease to improve. Intralesional hair follicle injections may be useful. Minoxidil preparations are modestly effective. L-Cysteine-containing shampoos may also be useful.

Other Manifestations

Lupus urticaria responds to steroids, antimalarials, H_1 and H_2 histamine blockers, and cyclosporine.

Lupus profundus is managed with local injections and antimalarials. Bullous lupus is frequently responsive to dapsone.

Lupus pemphigoid should be treated with mycophenolate mofetil.

Cutaneous vasculitis responds to corticosteroids. Colchicine or dapsone may be helpful.

The first-line treatment for Raynaud's phenomenon is cold avoidance, biofeedback, and cold-protection measures (e.g., gloves, mittens). Medication is used if the vasospasm is painful or there are skin ulcerations. Calcium channel blockers, especially nifedipine (30 to 90 mg/day), are the intervention of choice. If this class of drugs is not effective or is poorly tolerated, the following classes of drugs can be added to calcium channel blockers or used as monotherapy in the following order: nitroglycerin paste, 5-phosphodiesterase inhibitors (e.g., sildenafil), vasodilators (e.g., minoxidil), and α-blockers (e.g., α-methyldopa). Some angiotensin-converting enzyme inhibitors are minimally effective. Raynaud's activity does not correlate with disease activity.

Digital vasculitis can lead to gangrene. Patients are given Raynaud's remedies in addition to corticosteroids and immunosuppressive therapies. Resistant cases also benefit from prostaglandin-blocking agents (e.g., alprostadil infusions) and digital sympathectomy.

Musculoskeletal

Management of the synovitis of lupus arthritis depends on the degree of inflammation and whether or not erosions are present. NSAIDs or salicylates are helpful. Hydroxychloroquine is ameliorative. Most cases respond to 10 mg or less of prednisone daily. In doses similar to those used in RA, methotrexate (10 to 15 mg weekly with 1 mg of folic acid daily) or leflunomide (20 mg/day after a loading dose) is usually effective within 30 days. Tumor necrosis factor inhibitors can be used if erosions are present and patients do not have antibodies to double-stranded DNA. Abatacept, azathioprine, or rituximab represent effective alternative therapies.

Lupus myositis responds to prednisone 20 mg/day for several weeks if serum creatine phosphokinase levels are less than 500 IU. More active myositis is approached with higher doses of corticosteroids in combination with methotrexate, azathioprine, or rituximab.

Pulmonary

Nonscarring *pleuritic* pain in SLE responds to high-dose NSAIDs or short courses of moderate-dose corticosteroids. Higher doses of corticosteroids with either antimalarial or immunosuppressive maintenance are used in individuals with *pleural effusions*. Refractory cases can be managed with a pleurodesis or pleurectomy.

Acute lupus pneumonitis is fatal unless patients are given high doses of corticosteroids acutely.

The treatment of *interstitial lung disease* depends upon its level of activity. If it is deemed to have a reversible component, corticosteroids are usually initiated along with immunosuppressive therapy such as cyclophosphamide or azathioprine.

Pulmonary hemorrhage has a very high mortality rate. Those who have the greatest chance for survival include patients who have received pulse corticosteroids, cyclophosphamide with or without plasmapheresis.

Pulmonary hypertension mandates aggressive vigilance and treatment when pulmonary pressures rise above 50 mmHg. Vasodilators and calcium channel blockers may be useful in mild cases, but progressive pressure elevations usually mandate endothelin receptor antagonists, 5-phosphodiesterase blockers (e.g., sildenafil), or prostaglandin E_1/prostacyclin derivatives. Infrequently, pulmonary hypertension is a manifestation of vasculitis and responds to corticosteroids. Heart-lung transplantation may be advisable in advanced, medication-unresponsive patients.

Cardiac

Pericarditis is managed similarly to pleurisy. Pericardial tamponade or hemodynamically compromising effusions are uncommon, but a pericardiocentesis can be of diagnostic and therapeutic value.

Myocardial dysfunction in SLE is treated with inotropic agents, β-blockers, diuretics, and angiotensin-converting enzyme inhibitors. Acute myocarditis responds to 1 mg/kg/day prednisone for several weeks.

Libman-Sacks endocarditis warrants more vigilance than medication therapy. Patients with this manifestation should be on daily low-dose aspirin, have dental prophylaxis, and be considered for platelet antagonists and possibly anticoagulation, depending on their antiphospholipid antibody profile.

Lupus patients with *hypertension* respond to most antihypertensives, but renal impairment plays a bigger role in this occurrence. Also, some antihypertensives have a sulfa component, which could be problematic.

Microvascular angina is treated with beta blockers and nitrates.

Nervous System

Central nervous system vasculitis is over-diagnosed. When truly present, the best response rates have been reported among those receiving pulse doses of corticosteroids (e.g., 1 g of methylprednisolone intravenously for 3 days) followed by high doses of prednisone for at least a month. Traditionally, patients do well with 750 mg/m^2 monthly of intravenous cyclophosphamide for 6 months. Maintenance therapy after this is usually not necessary. Patients who fail to quickly respond often benefit from the addition of a 60 mL/kg plasmapheresis for several days. Recent reports have also suggested that rituximab or intrathecal methotrexate can be beneficial. *Antiphospholipid syndrome* patients should not be given corticosteroids unless they have the "catastrophic antiphospholipid syndrome" subset or clear-cut evidence for systemic inflammation. Stroke patients should be anticoagulated with heparin followed by warfarin while the source of the process is being worked up.

The management of the *dysautonomic* syndromes of SLE (e.g., lupus headache, cognitive dysfunction) is similar. Anti-inflammatory medicines are not overly beneficial; anxiety reduction, biofeedback, cognitive-behavioral therapy, psychotropic medications, and antimalarials are the treatments of choice. Vasodilators are useful in selected circumstances. Corticosteroids should be avoided if there is no evidence for vasculitis or inflammation (see Table 11.4).

Nephritis

Renal involvement in SLE is best assessed with a kidney biopsy. Adjunctive measures include monitoring blood pressure; treating nephrosis with diuretics as needed; and low-protein, -salt, or -fat diets as indicated, as well as screening for and managing electrolyte imbalances.[4,5]

Proliferative nephritis is associated with a high probability for evolving end-stage renal disease at 10 years. The National Institutes of Health protocol

---

Table 11.4 Examples of management options for nervous system lupus

1. Rule out fibromyalgia, infection, or medication reaction-causing symptoms
2. Cerebral vasculitis: High-dose corticosteroids, cyclosphosphamide; rituximab, apheresis for selected cases; anticonvulsants and antipsychotic regimens as needed
3. Thromboembolic event due to antiphospholipid syndrome: Platelet antagonists, anticoagulation
4. Lupus headache/cognitive dysfunction (vasculopathy, not vasculitis): Antimalarials, psychotropics, cognitive-behavioral therapy, anxiety reduction measures, biofeedback, calcium channel blockers
5. Chronic organic brain syndrome: Emotional support, anticonvulsants if needed
6. Cryoglobulinemia or hyperviscosity: Steroids, apheresis, immune suppressive regimens
7. Thrombotic thrombocytopenia purpura: Apheresis, rituximab
8. Peripheral nervous system lupus: Steroids, intravenous immune globulin, gabapentin, rituximab or cyclophosphamide
9. Posterior reversible encephalopathy syndrome: Control blood pressure
10. Pseudotumor cerebri: Lumbar puncture
11. Lupus sclerosis: Multiple sclerosis regimens

used by most lupologists for the past 20 years involves giving 1 mg/kg/day of corticosteroids for 4 to 6 weeks, followed by tapering to a maintenance dose of 10 mg/day for at least 2 years. Concurrently, patients are also given intravenous cyclophosphamide monthly (750/m²) for 6 months followed by retreatment every 1 to 3 months for up to 3 years. One-third have a complete remission on this schedule, one-third respond at first but relapse, and one-third have no response. Recently, many centers have begun adding mycophenolate mofetil or azathioprine at 4 to 6 months in lieu of continuing cyclophosphamide. Infertility associated with cyclophosphamide can be attenuated by the use of leuprolide (Leupron), 3.75 mg subcutaneously (SC), 2 weeks before each chemotherapy dose. A pivotal trial comparing cyclophosphamide with mycophenolate mofetil for induction showed them to be equal in efficacy; however, patients with crescentic, aggressive nephritis were excluded. Pulse steroids or apheresis can be used short term for acute flares Mycophenolate is superior to azathioprine for maintenance or improvement.[6] Several biologicals are being studied in clinical trials for proliferative disease. Recent American College of Rheumatology guidelines for managing nephritis have been published and are summarized in Figure 11.3.

Membranous nephritis follows a slower, more indolent course, except that more patients are nephrotic and develop renal vein thrombosis. The above

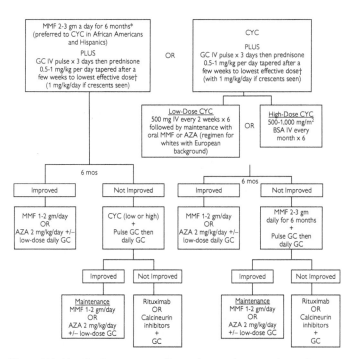

Figure 11.3 Algorithm for managing proliferative lupus nephritis according to the American College of Rheumatology guidelines.

regimens have been used successfully in these circumstances; however, there is evidence that cyclosporine may be effective and that some patients do not need any anti-inflammatory treatment (see Table 11.4).

Hemic-Lymphatic System

Diffuse adenopathy is generally quite responsive to moderate-dose corticosteroids.

Hemolytic anemia responds to high doses of steroids very slowly, and they may have to be given for several months before tapering. Response rates have been disappointing. Cyclophosphamide, azathioprine, or rituximab is usually added to the regimen.

The decision to treat *idiopathic thrombocytopenic purpura* (ITP) depends on the patient's platelet counts. No special treatment is required if the count is above 100,000/mm^3. Counts between 60,000 and 99,000/mm^3 are only treated if there is active inflammation evident outside the hemic-lymphatic system. Patients with counts less than 60,000/mm^3 are usually treated with corticosteroids. Cyclophosphamide, azathioprine, danocrine, or rituximab can be quite efficacious corticosteroid adjuncts. Intravenous immunoglobulin transiently raises platelet counts. Splenectomy is curative of ITP in 60% of medication-resistant cases.

Thrombotic thrombocytopenic purpura (TTP) is fatal in up to half of all cases. Plasma exchange is lifesaving; there is some evidence that rituximab is helpful as well.

Most of the agents commonly prescribed in SLE are summarized in Table 11.5.

Alternative and Complementary Medicine

In the United States, 40% of the population uses complementary and alternative medicines, spending $27 billion a year. Lupus patients tend to use four types of approaches[3]:

1. *Manipulative, physical, and manual therapies.* These include acupuncture, Pilates, chiropractics, reflexology, tai chi, and yoga. Any technique that strengthens muscles and promotes aerobic conditioning is acceptable, and some diminish pain.

2. *Methods that promote relaxation, cognitive improvement, and greater disease understanding.* Aromatherapy, biofeedback, cognitive-behavioral therapy, guided imagery, meditation, and prayer are examples of these methods. Evidence-based studies involving lupus have demonstrated that any activity that works with the mind–body connection, decreases anxiety, and promotes restful sleep is usually helpful.

3. *Detoxification regimens* such as colonic irrigation, magnet therapy, or chelation therapies are unproven in lupus and potentially dangerous.

4. *Herbal, dietary, and neutroceutical approaches* include homeopathic remedies, lifestyle diets (e.g., elemental, hypoallergenic, fasting, elimination), folk remedies, and vitamin regimens. Some supplements might be beneficial, but the majority are unproven (see Table 11.6).

Table 11.5 Drugs frequently used to manage systemic lupus erythematosus (SLE)

1. NSAIDs	Used for fever, headache, serositis, arthralgia/arthritis, myalgia, fever
	Naproxen has the best efficacy/safety profile in doses of 500 mg BID
	Gastroprotective measures may be advisable with chronic use
2. Antimalarials	Hydroxychloroquine is FDA approved for SLE and rheumatoid arthritis (RA)
	Has disease-modifying properties and is steroid sparing
	Useful in patients with antiphospholipid syndrome, Sjögren's
	Decreases cholesterol levels
	Indicated in 90% of lupus patients in doses of 5 mg/kg/day
	Not tolerated in 10%; retinal examinations should be performed annually
	Quinacrine or chloroquine can be used for resistant skin lesions
3. Corticosteroids	Approved by the FDA for SLE
	Induction therapy for organ-threatening disease is 1 mg/kg/day of prednisone equivalent for at least 4 to 6 weeks, followed by tapering
	Non-organ-threatening disease responds to 0.25 mg/kg/day or less
	Steroid-sparing alternatives (immunosuppressants) should be introduced with chronic use
4. Immunosuppressants	i. Methotrexate: FDA approved for RA, indicated for synovitis and some rashes in RA doses
	ii. Azathioprine: FDA approved for RA, steroid sparing in patients with organ-threatening disease, dosed at 100 to 150 mg/day
	iii. Cyclophosphamide: Effective for nephritis and CNS vasculitis, helpful in selected patients with organ-threatening disease. Numerous toxicities.
	iv. Mycophenolate mofetil: Effective for nephritis; 20% have gastrointestinal tolerance issues; unproven for other aspects of the disease
	v. Leflunomide: FDA approved for RA; effective for synovitis in RA doses
	vi. Cyclosporin: FDA approved for RA; may be useful for membranous nephritis, red cell hypoplasia, and lupus urticaria in RA doses
5. Biologicals	i. Anti-TNF blockers: FDA approved for RA; can be used in selected lupus patients; issues include disease exacerbation or rash, autoantibody development, infection risk in RA doses
	ii. Rituximab: FDA approved for RA; reports suggest efficacy for organ-threatening complications in RA doses
	iii. Tocilizumab: Promising trials for lupus underway
	iv. Abatacept: Trials in progress for nephritis and may help arthritis
	v. Belimumab: Approved for active autoantibody positive SLE not responsive to community standard of care

Table 11.6 Herbs studied for lupus, fibromyalgia, and other rheumatic disorders using evidence-based principles

Herb	Comments
Alfalfa	L-canavanine in alfalfa sprouts may flare lupus
Capsicum	Capsaicin is a proven topical analgesic in osteoarthritis
Echinacea	Reports of lupus flares from immune stimulation
Gingko biloba	May help cognitive impairment
Green tea extract	Reports of improvement in collagen-induced arthritis models
L-tryptophan	Sleep aid; contaminants can cause a scleroderma-like illness
St. John's wort	A natural serotonin booster
T wilfordii	Thunder-god vine; used in China for lupus, very potent
Valerian root	May improve sleep

References

1. Wallace DJ, Hahn BH. Section 6: The management of lupus. In: DJ Wallace, BH Hahn, eds. *Dubois' Lupus Erythematosus and related disorders.* 78h ed. Philadelphia, PA: Elsevier 2013:582–658.

2. Canadian Cooperative Study Group. A randomized study of the effect of withdrawing hydroxychloroquine sulfate in systemic lupus erythematosus. The Canadian Hydroxychloroquine Study Group. *N Engl J Med.* 1991;324:150–154.

3. Balow JE, Austin HA 3rd, Tsokos GC, Antonovych TT, Steinberg AD, Klippel JH. NIH conference. Lupus nephritis. *Ann Intern Med.* 1987;106:79–94.

4. Ernst E. Musculoskeletal conditions and complementary/alternative medicine. *Best Pract Res Clin Rheumatol.* 2004;18(4):539–556.

5. Hahn BH, Mc Mahon MA, Wilkinson A, et al, American College of Rheumatology guidelines for screening, treatment and management of lupus nephritis. *Arthritis Care Res (Hoboken).* 2012;64:797–808.

6. Dooley MA, Jayne D, Ginzler EM, et al. Mycophenolate versus azathioprine as maintenance therapy for lupus nephritis. *N Engl J Med.* 2011;365:1886–1895.

7. Wallace DJ, Gudsoorkar VS, Weisman MH et al, New insights into mechanisms of therapeutic effects of antimalarial agents in SLE. *Nature Rev Rheumatol.* 2012;8:522–533.

8. Marmor MF, Kellner U, Lai TY, Lyons JS, et al. Revised recommendations on screening for chloroquine and hydroxychloroquine retinopathy. *Ophthalmology.* 2011;118:415–422.

Chapter 12

Economic Impact and Disability Issues

Lupus costs the American public approximately $20 billion a year in lost wages, disability, hospitalizations, medical visits, and medication (Fig. 12.1). Direct costs account for one-third, and indirect costs two-thirds, of this amount.[1,3]

The overwhelming majority of lupus patients with non-organ-threatening disease are employed full time, while 50% with organ involvement are disabled[4] (Fig. 12.2). U.S. government guidelines are written in a way that makes it relatively easy for the latter group to obtain Medicare insurance and receive Social Security disability payments if they have contributed money to the system. Patients with cutaneous disease should avoid outdoor jobs, cold avoidance is desirable if Raynaud's phenomenon is present, and those with musculoskeletal impairments may benefit from vocational rehabilitation and an ergonomic evaluation of their work station. Flexible hours are often desirable to accommodate fatigue and pacing issues. Lupus patients are said to be "differently abled." They should be honest with their employer and emphasize what they can do, as opposed to what duties they are unable to perform. Part-time employment is possible for many lupus patients. Total permanent disability is not to be taken lightly. Disabled patients tend to be less independent, less socially interactive, and more depressed, and to have less self-esteem.[2]

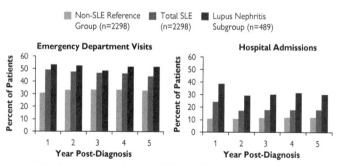

Figure 12.1 Emergency Room Visits by SLE Patients.[3]

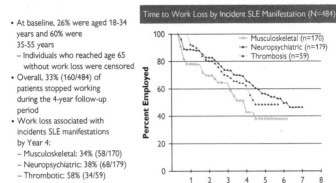

Work Loss Is a Common Consequence of SLE

- At baseline, 26% were aged 18-34 years and 60% were 35-55 years
  - Individuals who reached age 65 without work loss were censored
- Overall, 33% (160/484) of patients stopped working during the 4-year follow-up period
- Work loss associated with incidents SLE manifestations by Year 4:
  - Musculoskeletal: 34% (58/170)
  - Neuropsychiatric: 38% (68/179)
  - Thrombotic: 58% (34/59)

Yelin E, et al. *Arthritis Care Res (Hoboken)*. 2012; 64:169–175.

Figure 12.2 Disability Among SLE Patients.

References

1. Sutcliffe N, Clarke AE, Taylor R, et al. Total cost and predictors in patients with systemic lupus erythematosus. *Rheumatology*. 2001;40:37–47.

2. Yelin E, Trupin L, Katz P, et al. Work dynamics among persons with systemic lupus erythematosus. *Arthritis Rheum*. 2007;57(1):56–63.

3. Li T, Carls GS, Panopalis P, et al. Long term medical costs and resource utilization in systemis lupus erythematosus and lupus nephritis: a five-year analysis of a large Medicaid population. *Arthritis Rheum*. 2009;61:755–763.

4. Yelin E, Tonner C, Trupin L, et al. Longitudinal study of the impact of incident organ manifestations and increased disease activity on work loss among persons with systemic lupus erythematosus. *Arthritis Rheum*. 2012;64:169–175.

Chapter 13

Prognosis

Prior to the availability of corticosteroids and immunosuppressive therapy, which became widely accessible after 1948, half of persons with lupus died within two years, and half survived. This generally demarcated organ- versus non-organ-threatening disease. Table 13.1 shows the gradual improvement in outcome over the past 60 years. Currently, most patients with systemic lupus erythematosus survive at least 20 years,[1] although their quality of life is not always optimal. Historically, 40% of deaths in lupus patients with serious disease were from inflammation and occurred within two years of diagnosis. Approximately 10% of deaths took place over the following 10 years. The remaining 40% of lupus patients died 12 to 25 years after diagnosis, mostly from infections and complications of chronic steroid therapy and immunosuppression. This "bimodal" curve has been altered in the past 10 years.[2] Death due to lupus during the first two years is becoming less common; individuals with serious SLE still have a 10- to 30-year shortened life expectancy due to complications of therapy.[3] Figure 13.1 summarizes the principal causes of death in SLE.[5,6]

Patients with drug-induced lupus, chronic cutaneous lupus, and non-organ-threatening SLE without antiphospholipid antibodies have a normal survival rate. The outcome of lupus patients depends on a variety of other factors (see Fig. 13.2): race; ethnicity; geography; access to health care; adherence to medication; gender; clinical and laboratory variables; treatment variables; presence of antiphospholipid syndrome; and attention to comorbidities such as accelerated atherogenesis, smoking cessation, weight reduction, patient education, and osteoporosis. Approximately 5% of persons with SLE experience spontaneous remission without treatment.

Over the past decade, a surprising number of approaches and interventions have been shown to improve the quality of life and outcome of patients with SLE without prescribing lupus medications.[4]

Table 13.1 Prognosis of lupus erythematosus

1. Normal life expectancy in >95% of patients:
   - Drug-induced lupus
   - Chronic cutaneous lupus
   - Non-organ-threatening systemic lupus erythematosus without antiphospholipid antibodies
2. Important benchmarks in 5- and 10-year survival rates for all SLE patients:

Study authors	Year	5 years	10 years
Merill and Shulman	1955	50%	
Estes and Christian	1971	77%	60%
Wallace and Dubois	1981	88%	79%
Reveille	1990	89%	83%
Urowitz and Gladman	1995	93%	85%
Recent studies	2000–2013	95%	90%

1. Only 75% with SLE survive 25 years in most centers with a diversity of patients.
2. Evolution of survival for patients with lupus nephritis:
   a. No survival to poor survival prior to widespread availability of dialysis since 1969
   b. Wallace and Dubois (1981): 60% 10-year survival rate (30% if nephritic)
   c. Esdaile (1989): 85% and 73% 5- and 10-year survival rates
   d. Work since 2000: Most live 10 years; high percentage succumb at 10 to 25 years

Bimodal Mortality

Early deaths:

• Renal involvement and high incidence of infection

Late deaths:

• High incidence of myocardial infarction (MI) due to atherosclerotic heart disease

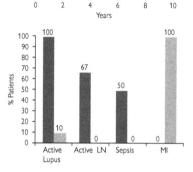

Figure 13.1 Early and late complications of systemic lupus erythematosus (SLE).
Source: Urowitz MB, Bookman AA, Koehler BE, Gordon DA, Smythe HA, Ogryzlo MA. The bimodal mortality pattern of systemic lupus erythematosus. Am J Med. 1976;60(2):221–225. Reprinted with permission. Elsevier, ©1976.

Cardiovascular Events, Malignancies, and Infections Are Among the Most Common Causes of Death in SLE

• A range of organ systems are implicated in SLE mortality
  – Mortality data from 9547 patients followed 1958–2001; total of 1255 deaths occured
  – Patients followed for 76,948 person-years
• Mortality rates were significantly higher for some of the most common causes of death than those seen in the general population
  – ~8x higher for renal causes
  – ~5x higher for infections
  – Almost 2x higher for heart disease

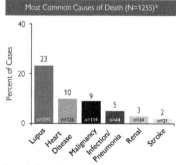

Bernatsky S, et al. Arthritis Rheum. 2006; 54:2550–2557.

Figure 13.2 Most common causes of death in SLE.

References

1. Abu-Shakra M, Urowitz MB, Gladman DD, et al. Mortality studies in systemic lupus erythematosus. Results from a single centre, 1. Causes of death. J Rheumatol. 1995;22:1259–1264.

2. Urowitz MB, Bookman AA, Koehler BE, et al. The bimodal mortality pattern of systemic lupus erythematosus. Am J Med. 1976;60:221–225.

3. Ward MM. Hospital experience and mortality in patients with systemic lupus erythematosus. Arthritis Rheum. 1999;42:891–898.

4. Wallace DJ. Viewpoint: improving the prognosis of SLE without prescribing lupus drugs and the primary care paradox. *Lupus*. 2008;17:91–92.

5. Bernatsky S, Boivin J, Manzi S, et al. Mortality in systemic lupus erythematosus. *Arthritis Rheum*. 2006;54:2550–2557.

6. Bernatsky S, Levy D, Ramsey-Goldman R, Gordon C, Rahman A, Clarke AE. Mortality in SLE. In: DJ Wallace and BH Hahn, eds. *Dubois' Lupus Erythematosus and Related Syndromes*, 8th ed.Philadelphia, PA: Elsevier; 2013:666–675.

Chapter 14

Experimental and Innovative Therapies

As of this writing, only one biological intervention (belimumab) has been approved for systemic lupus erythematosus.[1] Numerous agents are in clinical trials and are summarized here. The landscape is continuously changing.[1] The reader is referred to the www.clinicaltrials.gov Web site for up-to-date information.

Targeted Therapies Used in SLE Currently Approved by the FDA

Agents that block *anti-TNF* (e.g., remicade, trade name Infliximab; etanercept, Enbrel; adalimumab, Humira) have been available since 1998 and are widely prescribed for rheumatoid arthritis, inflammatory bowel disease, psoriasis, psoriatic arthritis, uveitis, and for juvenile inflammatory arthritis. Thousands of lupus patients have used these drugs. A summary of experience suggests that patients with prominent inflammatory arthritis (swollen joints) may do well with anti-TNFs, especially if there is a lupus/rheumatoid overlap. However, some individuals experience increases in anti-DNA, ANA, and anticardiolipin antibodies as well as more infections.

Rituximab (Rituxan) is a B-cell depletion drug that is given intravenously 1–2 weeks apart every 6 months or as needed. It is generally well tolerated but can have major side effects, including being associated with serious infections. Controlled trials using this drug for severe lupus and lupus nephritis had negative results, but study designs were controversial. There is a wealth of experience in case series demonstrating that lupus patients with severe arthritis, central nervous system vasculitis, low platelet counts, and hemolytic anemia do well with this agent[2] (See Table 14.1).

Abatacept (Orencia) inhibits the T-cell co-stimulatory pathway and is approved for rheumatoid arthritis. It can be given intravenously once a month or as a weekly injection. Abatacept is very well tolerated, but two controlled studies using it for SLE have had conflicting results. It may play a role in patients with serious SLE who would benefit from steroid and immune suppressive sparing approaches.[3]

Belimumab (Benlysta) blocks soluble B lymphocyte stimulator (BlyS) that increases inflammation, and is approved for patients with SLE who are antibody-positive with active disease in spite of receiving community standard of care therapy.[4] Given as an intravenous monthly after a loading period, belimumab starts working in 3–6 months. Studies have shown that it decreases

Table 14.1 Targets for new therapies in systemic lupus erythematosus

T cells	Abatacept; modified CD40L monoclonal antibody; ICOS inhibition
B cells, anti-dsDNA antibodies	Monoclonal antibodies to CD20 (rituxan), CD22 (epratuzumab); anti-BLyS TACI-Ig; BAFF-RFc (belimumab, tabalumab, blisbimod, actacicept)
Complement	Anti-C5a (eculizumab)
Cytokines	Monoclonal antibodies to IL-6R (tocilizumab), IL-6, IL-10, IL-17, IL-21
Promote regulatory cells	Expand CD4 + CD25+ cells, CD8 + CD28– cells
Inhibition of interferon, Toll receptors (innate immune system)	Anti-IFN-alpha (rontilizumab, sifilimumab); TLR7 and TLR9 antagonists
T cell regulation of autoantibody production, tolerogens	Peptides derived from nucleosomes, splicosome; SmAg Igs; 16/6 idiotype
Cell surface receptor activation inhibition	Syk-kinase inhibition, kinome directed therapies (tofacitinib), rapamycin

inflammatory levels and is steroid- and immune-suppressive sparing and also improves quality of life. Belimumab has an excellent safety profile and is very well tolerated (Fig. 14.1). We use it in patients who have active disease despite steroids and immune-suppressive therapies, or are intolerant to these interventions, or cannot take the usually efficacious doses of those agents.

Targeted Therapies Currently in Development

The principal approaches being studied are summarized in Table 14.1. None of the T cell approaches listed other that abatacept will be available for many

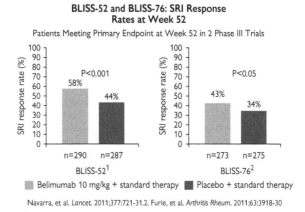

BLISS-52 and BLISS-76: SRI Response Rates at Week 52

Patients Meeting Primary Endpoint at Week 52 in 2 Phase III Trials

BLISS-52[1]: P<0.001, 58% (n=290), 44% (n=287)

BLISS-76[2]: P<0.05, 43% (n=273), 34% (n=275)

Belimumab 10 mg/kg + standard therapy   Placebo + standard therapy

Navarra, et al. *Lancet.* 2011;377:721-31.2. Furie, et al. *Arthritis Rheum.* 2011;63:3918-30

Figure 14.1 Efficacy of belimumab for SLE.

Table 14.2 Innovative approaches under study
1. T-cell vaccination
2. Agents that target chemokines
3. Peptide tolerogens to HLA molecules, Sm, and immunoglobulin
4. Promotion of T regulatory cells
5. Gene therapies
6. Upregulation of transforming growth factor-β
7. Targeting Fc receptors
8. Developing gene transcription regulators
9. Inhibition of interleukin-12, -15, -17, or -18
10. Induction of anergy in T helper cells
11. Mesenchymal stem cells
12. Inhibition of adhesion molecules
13. Inhibitor of co-stimulation (CD80 [AV1142742])
14. Targeting urinary cytokines
15. Epigenetics: histone deacetylase inhibition; promotion of methylation

years. Several agents that block BlyS or related compounds are in Phase II and Phase III trials. These include tabalumab, blisbimod, and atacicept. Epratuzumab is an anti-CD22 with novel mechanisms of action in addition to reduction in B cells (e.g., trogocytosis, internalization of cell signaling) and is currently in a Phase III trial. Eculizumab is already on the market for paroxysmal nocturnal hemoglobinuria and atypical hemolytic uremic syndrome and is promising for lupus. Cytokine inhibition via blockade of interleukin 6 is being studied by several companies and is already approved for rheumatoid arthritis. Targeting the innate immune system via interferon or Toll receptors is a focus of many initiatives. Small molecules that interfere with cell signaling are also promising, and one agent (tofacitinib) is already approved for rheumatoid arthritis.

It is highly likely that the management of lupus will be totally altered in the next five years, and the outcome, quality of life, and ultimate prognosis for persons with the disease will drastically change.

References

1. Wallace DJ. Ten developments in the use of biological for systemic lupus erythematosus. *Curr Rheumatol Rep.* 2013;15:337.

2. Merrill JT, Neuwelt CM, Wallace DJ, et al. Efficacy and safety of rituximab in moderately-to-severely active systemic lupus erythematosus: the randomized, double-blind, phase II/III systemic lupus erythematosus evaluation of rituximab trial. *Arthritis Rheum.* 2010;62:222.

3. Merrill JT, Borgos-Vargas R, Westhovens R, et al. The efficacy and safety of abatacept in patients with non-life-threatening manifestations of systemic lupus erythematosus: results of a twelve-month, multicenter, exploratory, phase IIb, randomized, double-blind, placebo-controlled trial. *Arthritis Rheum.* 2010;62:3077–3087.

4. Navarra SV, Guzman RM, Gallacher AE, et al.; BLISS-52 Study Group. Efficacy and safety of belimumab in patients with active systemic lupus erythematosus: a randomised, placebo-controlled, phase 3 trial. *Lancet.* 2011;377:721–731.

Glossary

ACR: The American College of Rheumatology, formerly known as the ARA (American Rheumatism Association). A professional association of 4,000 American rheumatologists, of whom 2,800 are board certified. Criteria, or definitions for many rheumatic diseases, are referred to as *ACR criteria*.

Acute: Coming on suddenly and of short duration.

Adenopathy: Swelling of lymph nodes.

Adrenal glands: Small organs located above the kidney that produce many hormones, including corticosteroids and epinephrine.

Albumin: Protein that circulates in the blood and carries materials to cells.

Albuminuria: Protein in urine.

Alopecia: Hair loss.

Analgesic: Drug that alleviates pain.

Anemia: Condition resulting from low red blood cell counts.

Antibodies
: Special protein substances made by the body's white blood cells for defense against bacteria and other foreign substances.

Anticentromere antibody: Antibody to a part of a cell's nucleus; associated with a form of scleroderma called CREST (see its listing).

Anticardiolipin antibody: Antiphospholipid antibody.

Anti-double-stranded DNA (anti-DNA): Antibodies to DNA; seen in half of those with systemic lupus; implies serious disease.

Anti-ENA: Old term for *extractable nuclear antibodies*, which largely consist of anti-Sm and anti-RNP antibodies.

Antigen: Substance that stimulates antibody formation; in lupus, this can be a foreign substance or a product of the patient's own body.

Anti-inflammatory: Agent that counteracts or suppresses inflammation.

Antimalarials: Drugs traditionally used to treat malaria that are helpful for lupus.

Antinuclear antibodies (ANA): Proteins in the blood that react with the nuclei of cells. Seen in 96% of those with SLE, in 5% of healthy individuals, and in most patients with autoimmune diseases.

Antiphospholipid antibodies: Antibodies to a constituent of cell membranes seen in one-third of those with SLE. In the presence of a co-factor, these antibodies can alter clotting and lead to strokes, blood clots, miscarriages, and low platelet counts. Also detected as the lupus anticoagulant.

Anti-RNP: Antibody to ribonucleoprotein. Seen in SLE and mixed connective tissue disease.

Anti-Sm: Anti-Smith antibody; found only in lupus.

Anti-SSA: Ro antibody; associated with Sjögren's syndrome, sun sensitivity, neonatal lupus, and congenital heart block.

Anti-SSB: La antibody; almost always seen with anti-SSA.

Apheresis: See *Plasmapheresis*.

Apoptosis: Programmed cell death.

Artery: Blood vessel that transports blood from the heart to the tissues.

Arthralgia: Pain in a joint.

Arthritis: Inflammation of a joint.

Ascites: Abnormal collection of abdominal fluid.

Aspirin: Anti-inflammatory drug with pain-killing properties.

Atrophy: Thinning of a surface; a form of wasting.

Autoantibody: Antibody to one's own tissues or cells.

Autoimmunity: Allergy to one's own tissues.

Autoimmune hemolytic anemia: See *Hemolytic anemia*.

B lymphocyte or B cell: White blood cell that makes antibodies.

Biologics: Targeted immune therapies.

Biopsy: Removal of a bit of tissue for examination under the microscope.

Bursa: Sac of synovial fluid between tendons, muscles, and bones that promotes easier movement.

Butterfly rash: Reddish facial eruption over the bridge of the nose and cheeks, resembling a butterfly in flight.

Capillaries: Small blood vessels connecting arteries and veins.

Cartilage: Tissue material covering bone. The nose, outer ears, and trachea consist primarily of cartilage.

Candida: A yeast.

Chronic: Persisting over a long period of time.

CNS: Central nervous system.

Collagen: Structural protein found in bone, cartilage, and skin.

Collagen vascular disease (also called *connective tissue disease*): Antibody-mediated inflammatory process of the connective tissues, especially the joints, skin, and muscle.

Congenital heart block: Dysfunction of the rate/rhythm conduction system in the fetal or infant heart.

Connective tissue: "Glue" that holds together muscles, skin, and joints.

Complement: Group of proteins that, when activated, promote and are consumed during inflammation.

Complete blood count (CBC): Blood test that measures the amounts of red blood cells, white blood cells, and platelets in the body.

Corticosteroid: Any natural anti-inflammatory hormone made by the adrenal cortex; also can be made synthetically.

Cortisone: Synthetic corticosteroid.

Creatinine: Breakdown product of creatine, a muscle component.

Creatinine clearance: A 24-hour urine collection test that measures kidney function.

CREST syndrome: Form of limited scleroderma characterized by C (calcium deposits under the skin), R (Raynaud's phenomenon), E (esophageal dysfunction), S (sclerodactyly, or tight skin), and T (telangiectasia, a rash).

Crossover syndrome: Autoimmune process that has features of more than one rheumatic disease (e.g., lupus and scleroderma).

Cryoglobulins: Protein complexes circulating in the blood that are precipitated by cold.

Cutaneous: Relating to the skin.

Cytokines: Group of chemicals that signal cells to perform certain actions.

Dermatologist: Physician specializing in skin diseases.

Dermatomyositis: Autoimmune process directed against muscles and associated with skin rashes.

Discoid lupus: Thick, plaquelike rash seen in 20% of those with SLE. If the patient has the rash but not SLE, he or she is said to have *cutaneous* (discoid) lupus erythematosus.

Diuretics: Medications that increase the body's ability to rid itself of fluids.

DNA: Deoxyribonucleic acid; the body's building blocks; a molecule responsible for the production of all the body's proteins.

Dysphagia: Difficulty swallowing.

Ecchymosis: Purplish patch caused by oozing of blood into the skin.

Edema: Swelling caused by retention of fluid.

ELISA (enzyme-linked immunosorbent assay): Very sensitive blood test for detecting the presence of autoantibodies.

Enzyme: Protein that accelerates chemical reactions.

Epigenetics: The ability of the environment to alter gene expression.

Erythema: Reddish hue.

Erythematous: Having a reddish hue.

Estrogen: Female hormone produced by the ovaries.

Exacerbations: Symptoms reappear; a flare.

False-positive serological test for syphilis: Blood test revealing an antibody that may be found in patients with syphilis and that gives false-positive results in 15% of patients with SLE. Associated with the lupus anticoagulant and antiphospholipid antibodies.

FANA: Another term for ANA.

Fibrositis, or fibromyalgia: Pain amplification syndrome characterized by fatigue, a sleep disorder, and tender points in the soft tissues; can be caused by steroids and mistaken for lupus, although 20% of those with lupus have fibrositis.

Flare: Symptoms reappear; another word for exacerbation.

Gene: Consisting of DNA, it is the basic unit of inherited information in our cells.

Glomerulonephritis: Inflammation of the glomerulus of the kidney; seen in one-third of patients with lupus.

Hematocrit: Measurement of red blood cell levels. Low levels produce anemia.

Hemoglobin: Oxygen-carrying protein of red blood cells. Low levels produce anemia.

Hemolytic anemia: Anemia caused by premature destruction of red blood cells due to antibodies to the red blood cell surface. Also called *autoimmune hemolytic anemia*.

Hepatitis: Inflammation of the liver.

HLA, or histocompatibility antigen: Molecules inside a macrophage that binds to an antigenic peptide. Controlled by genes on the sixth chromosome. They can amplify or perpetuate certain immune and inflammatory responses.

Hormones: Chemical messengers—including thyroid hormones, steroids, insulin, estrogen, progesterone, and testosterone—made by the body.

Immune complex: Antibody and antigen bound together.

Immunofluorescence: Means of detecting immune processes with a fluorescent stain and a special microscope.

Immunoglobulus: Protein fraction of serum responsible for antibody activity.

Immunity: Body's defense against foreign substances.

Immunosuppressant: Medication such as cyclophosphamide or azathioprine, which treats lupus by suppressing the immune system.

Inflammation: Swelling, heat, and redness resulting from the infiltration of white blood cells into tissues.

Interferon: Protein that fights infection but is inappropriately activated in lupus.

Kidney biopsy: Removal of a bit of kidney tissue for microscopic analysis.

La antibody: Also called anti-SSB; a Sjögren's antibody.

LE cell: Specific cell found in blood specimens of most lupus patients.

Ligament: Tether attaching bone to bone, providing stability.

Lupus anticoagulant: Means of detecting antiphospholipid antibodies from prolonged clotting times.

Lupus vulgaris: Tuberculosis of the skin; not related to systemic or discoid lupus.

Lymph: Fluid collected from tissues that flows through lymph nodes.

Lymphocyte: Type of white blood cell that fights infection and mediates the immune response.

Macrophage: Cell that kills foreign material and presents information to lymphocytes.

MHC: Major histocompatibility complex; in humans, it is the same as HLA.

Mixed connective tissue disease: Exists when a patient who carries the anti-RNP antibody has features of more than one autoimmune disease.

Natural killer cell: White blood cell that kills other cells.

Nephritis: Inflammation of the kidney.

Neutrophil: Granulated white blood cell involved in bacterial killing and acute inflammation.

NSAID: Nonsteroidal anti-inflammatory drug; agent that fights inflammation by blocking the actions of prostaglandin. Examples include aspirin, ibuprofen, and naproxen.

Nucleus: Center of a cell; contains DNA.

Orthopedic surgeon: Physician who operates on musculoskeletal structures.

Pathogenic: Causing disease or abnormal reactions.

Pathology: Abnormal cellular or anatomic features.

Pericardial effusion: Fluid around the sac of the heart.

Pericarditis: Inflammation of the pericardium.

Pericardium: Sac lining the heart.

Petechiae: Small red spots under the skin.

Photosensitivity: Sensitivity to ultraviolet light.

Plasma: Fluid portion of blood.

Plasmapheresis: Filtration of blood plasma through a machine to remove proteins that may aggravate lupus.

Platelet: Component of blood responsible for clotting.

Pleura: Sac lining the lung.

Pleural effusion: Fluid in the sac lining the lung.

Pleuritis: Irritation or inflammation of the lining of the lung.

Polyarteritis: Disease closely related to lupus featuring inflammation of medium-sized and small blood vessels.

Polymyalgia rheumatica: Autoimmune disease of the joints and muscles seen in older patients with high sedimentation rates who have severe aching in their shoulders, upper arms, hips, and upper legs.

Polymyositis: Autoimmune disease that targets muscles.

Prednisone; prednisolone: Synthetic steroids.

Protein: Collection of amino acids. Antibodies are proteins.

Proteinuria: Excess protein levels in the urine (also called *albuminuria*).

Pulse steroids: Very high doses of corticosteroids given intravenously over one to three days to critically ill patients.

Purpura: Hemorrhage into the skin.

Raynaud's disease: Isolated Raynaud's phenomenon; not part of any other disease.

Raynaud's phenomenon: Discoloration of the hands or feet (they turn blue, white, or red), especially with cold temperatures; a feature of an autoimmune disease.

RBC: Red blood cell.

Remission: Quiet period free from symptoms but not necessarily representing true resolution of the disease.

Rheumatic disease: Any of 150 disorders affecting the immune or musculoskeletal systems; about 30 of these are also autoimmune.

Rheumatoid arthritis: Chronic disease of the joints marked by inflammatory changes in the joint-lining membranes, which may give positive results on tests of rheumatoid factor and ANA.

Rheumatoid factor: Autoantibodies that react with IgG; seen in most patients with rheumatoid arthritis and 25% of those with SLE.

Rheumatologist: Internal medicine specialist who has completed at least a two-year fellowship studying rheumatic diseases (see *Rheumatic disease*).

Ro antibody: See *Anti-SSA*.

Salicylates: Aspirin-like drugs.

Scleroderma: Autoimmune disease featuring rheumatoid-type inflammation, tight skin, and vascular problems (e.g., *Raynaud's*).*Sedimentation rate*: Test that measures the precipitation of red cells in a column of blood; high rates usually indicate increased disease activity.

Serum: Clear liquid portion of the blood remaining after the removal of clotting factors.

Sjögren's syndrome: Dry eyes, dry mouth, and arthritis observed with most autoimmune disorders or by itself (primary Sjögren's).

Steroids: Usually a shortened term for corticosteroids, which are anti-inflammatory hormones produced either by the adrenal cortex or synthetically.

STS: Serological test for syphilis.

Symptoms: Changes from usual or healthy conditions that patients feel.

Synovial fluid: Joint fluid.

Synovitis: Inflammation of the tissues lining a joint.

Synovium: Tissue that lines a joint.

Systemic: Pertaining to or affecting the body as a whole.

T cell: Lymphocyte responsible for immunological memory.

Tendon: Structures that attach muscle to bone.

Temporal arteritis: Inflammation of the temporal artery (located in the scalp) associated with high sedimentation rates, systemic symptoms, and sometimes loss of vision.

Thrombocytopenia: Low platelet count.

Thymus: Gland in the neck area responsible for immunological maturity.

Titer: Amount of a substance, such as ANA.

Tolerance: Failure to make antibodies to an antigen.

Toll receptor: Part of the innate immune system that acts as a form of pattern recognition for the cell.

UCTD: Undifferentiated connective tissue disease; features of autoimmunity in a patient who does not meet the established criteria for lupus, rheumatoid arthritis, scleroderma, or inflammatory myositis.

Urinalysis: Analysis of urine.

Urine, 24-hour collection: Collection of all urine passed in a 24-hour period; the urine is examined for protein and creatinine to determine how well the kidneys are functioning.

Urticaria: Hives.

UV light: Ultraviolet light. Its spectrum includes UVA (320 to 400 nanometers [nm]), UVB (290 to 320 nm), and UVC (200 to 290 nm) wavelengths.

Uremia: Marked kidney insufficiency, frequently necessitating dialysis.

Vasculitis: Inflammation of the blood vessels.

WBC: White blood cell.

Appendix

Lupus Resource Materials

What organizations provide patient support in the United States? (Many such organizations exist; only those with a budget of over $1 million are listed.)

1. American Autoimmune Related Diseases Association (AARDA), 22100 Gratiot Avenue, E. Detroit, MI 48021, 1-810-776-3900 (national office); 750 17th Street, NW, Suite 1100, Washington, DC 20006, 1-202-466-8511. Web site: http://www.aarda.org

2. Arthritis Foundation, P.O. Box 7669, Atlanta, GA 30357, 1-800-283-7800. There are 56 U.S. chapters that provide research monies, publish literature, and offer patient support for arthritis and related conditions such as lupus. Web site: http://www.arthritis.org

3. Lupus Foundation of America, Inc. (LFA), 2000 L Street NW, Suite 710, Washington, DC 20036, 1-202-349-1155 or 1-800-558-0121 (Spanish line, 1-800-558-0123). With 50 chapters and 220 support groups in 32 states, the LFA is the nation's leading nonprofit voluntary health organization dedicated to finding the cause and cure for lupus. Web site: http://www.lupus.org

4. SLE Foundation, 300 Seventh Avenue, #1701, New York, NY 10001, 1-212-685-4118 or 1-800-74-LUPUS. Web site: http://www.lupusny.org

In addition to the above, where else can reliable information about lupus be obtained?

5. American College of Rheumatology (ACR) and Association of Rheumatology Health Professionals (ARHP), 1800 Century Place, Suite 250, Atlanta, GA 30345, 1-404-633-3777. This is the professional organization to which nearly all American and many international rheumatologists belong. Web site: http://www.rheumatology.org

6. National Institute of Arthritis and Musculoskeletal and Skin Diseases (NIAMS), Bldg. 31, Room 4C02, 31 Center Drive, MSC 2350, Bethesda, MD 20892, 1-301-496-8190. Toll free: 877-22NIAMS. Part of the National Institutes of Health, NIAMS funds nearly $100 million in lupus research each year at the Bethesda campus and elsewhere in the country. Web site: http://www.niams.nih.gov

In addition to the above, what other organizations fund lupus research? (Many such organizations exist; this list is restricted to those that give more than $1 million a year to lupus-related research at more than one institution.)

1. Alliance for Lupus Research, 28 West 44th Street, Suite 501, New York, NY 10036, 1-212-218-2840. Toll free: 1-800-5580121. This organization

was founded in 1999 with the mission to prevent, treat, and cure lupus through medical research. Web site: http://www.lupusresearch.org/index.html

2. Lupus Research Institute, 350 Seventh Avenue, #1701, New York NY 10001, 1-212-812-9881. The Institute was founded in 2000 to provide funding to novel research and clinically innovative lupus research projects. Web site: http://www.lupusresearchinstitute.org

3. Rheumatology Research Foundation of the American College of Rheumatology, 2200 Lake Boulevard NE, Atlanta, GA 30319, 1-800-346-4753. The research funding arm of the ACR provides money for rheumatology training and research programs that are vital to the care of patients suffering from rheumatic diseases. Web site: http://www.rheumatology.org/ref

How can I find out about lupus support outside the United States?

1. Lupus Europe. Most efforts in Europe are coordinated through a central office. Twenty-three affiliate groups are located in Belgium, Finland, France, Germany, Great Britain, Iceland, Ireland, Israel, Italy, the Netherlands, Norway, Portugal, Spain, Sweden, and Switzerland. E-mail: Tony Bonello; Web site: http://www.lupus-europe.org

2. Lupus Canada (the national organization), 3555 14th Avenue, Unit #3, Markham, Ontario L3R 0H5, Canada, 1-905-513-0004 or toll-free in Canada, 1-800-661-1468. Web site: http://www.lupuscanada.org (in French and English)

3. Panamerican League of Associations for Rheumatology. Comprises the scientific societies of rheumatology health professionals and rheumatic patient association in all the Americas.

Which organizations serve patients with lupus-related disorders?

1. Fibromyalgia Network, P.O. Box 31750, Tucson, AZ 85751-1750, 1-520-290-5508 or 1-800-853-2929. This organization supports research through the American Fibromyalgia Syndrome Association. Web site: http://www.fmnetnews.com

2. Scleroderma Foundation, 300 Rosewood Drive, #105, Danvers, MA 01923, 1-978-463-5843 or 1-800-722-4673. Web site: http://www.scleroderma.org.

3. Sjögren's Syndrome Foundation, 6707 Democracy Blvd, #325, Bethesda, MD 20817. Toll-free: 800-475-6473. Web site: http://www.sjogrens.org

What about rheumatology or lupus textbooks?

1. R. G. Lahita, G. Tsokos, J. Buyon, T. Koike, *Systemic Lupus Erythematosus*, 5th edition (Philadelphia: Academic Press, 2010).

2. D. J. Wallace, *Lupus* (New York: Oxford University Press, 2013).

3. D. J. Wallace and B. H. Hahn, *Dubois' Lupus Erythematosus*, 8th edition (Elsevier, 2013). The definitive text on the topic.

The best general rheumatology textbooks are as follows:

1. G. S. Firestein, R. C. Budd, E. D. Harris, Jr., et al., *Kelley's Textbook of Rheumatology*, 8th edition (Philadelphia: WB Saunders, 2008, two-volume set).
2. M. C. Hochberg, A. J. Silman, J. S. Smolen, M. E. Weinblatt, and M. H. Weisman, editors, *Rheumatology*, 5th edition, 2-volume set (Philadelphia: Elsevier, 2010).

How can I find another good book for lupus patients?

Over 200 books have been published that are aimed at lupus patients. They vary widely in their quality, focus, and expertise. A few simple rules will help in navigating Amazon, Barnes & Noble, or other listings.

1. Avoid all books that have "cure" in the title.
2. Individual testimonials can be compelling but are only occasionally applicable to the reader; no two lupus cases or circumstances are the same.
3. Books endorsed by the Arthritis Foundation, Lupus Foundation of America, or the SLE Foundation have been peer-reviewed by experts and generally are of superior quality.
4. Try to find books written by an M.D. who is involved in lupus research or patient care, especially if they are the first-listed author. Some efforts have an introduction or foreword by a lupus specialist and the reader can be misled from the book jacket to believe that the specialist actually wrote the book.
5. Avoid books more than 10 years old; the advice may be outdated or no longer valid.
6. New books are appearing all the time; consult the above-listed Web sites of lupus support organizations for updated listings.
7. There is no proven lupus diet or alternative therapy regimen. This is a serious disorder; consult your lupus specialist before embarking on any of these regimens.

Index